Maximize *Your* Healing Power

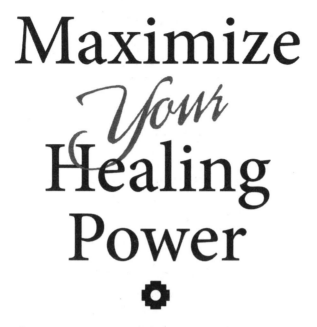

Shamanic Healing Techniques to Overcome Your Health Challenges

Sharon E. Martin, M.D., Ph.D.

FINDHORN PRESS

Findhorn Press
One Park Street
Rochester, Vermont 05767
www.findhornpress.com

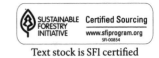

Text stock is SFI certified

Findhorn Press is a division of Inner Traditions International

---

Disclaimer

The information in this book is given in good faith and is neither intended to diagnose any physical or mental condition nor to serve as a substitute for informed medical advice or care. Please contact your health professional for medical advice and treatment. Neither author nor publisher can be held liable by any person for any loss or damage whatsoever which may arise from the use of this book or any of the information therein.

Cataloging-in-Publication data for this title is available from the Library of Congress

ISBN 978-1-64411-660-9 (print)
ISBN 978-1-64411-661-6 (ebook)

Printed and bound in the United States by Lake Book Manufacturing, LLC
The text stock is SFI certified. The Sustainable Forestry Initiative® program promotes sustainable forest management.

10 9 8 7 6 5 4 3 2 1

Edited by Nicky Leach
Illustrations by Sachin Vishwa and Ariane Yana Factor (chacana cover & interior)
Text design and layout by Richard Crookes
This book was typeset in Adobe Garamond Pro

To send correspondence to the author of this book, mail a first-class letter to the author c/o Inner Traditions • Bear & Company, One Park Street, Rochester, VT 05767, USA and we will forward the communication, or contact the author directly at **https://drsharonmartin.com**.

Maximize Your Healing Power

"One of the leading emerging voices in the energy healing field, Dr. Sharon Martin is both a shaman—one who enters the energy field to facilitate healing—and a board-certified internal medicine physician. Having experienced energy healing and other dimensions since an early age, she is uniquely equipped to present an integrated path that includes both approaches. Martin might order conventional Western medical tests for a patient and then might equally investigate a patient's soul contracts and energy patterns. She calls this 'Maximum Medicine.' The shamanic perspective is that the soul contracts with which you came into this life aren't static. The book includes many invitations to self-inquiry and shamanic exercises, one of which encourages you to change the rules of the game. A superb contribution to the new paradigm in healing, *Maximize Your Healing Power* is highly recommended for anyone seeking to understand every dimension of their health and maximize their vitality."

— **Dawson Church, Ph.D.,** researcher, founder of the National Institute for Integrative Healthcare (NIIH), and author of *The Genie in Your Genes* and *Mind to Matter*

"Dr. Martin, through personal stories, shows that Western medicine can blend with shamanic practices to give a more holistic approach to healing. She outlines a clear step-by-step process, through guided meditation, to take control of the healing journey. I recommend this book for any patient who wants to go deeper into healing and also for medical students and residents who want to step outside the box and see the patient as a whole person."

— **Janene Glyn, M.D.,** hospital physician, Altru medical school faculty, and shamanic practitioner

"*Maximize Your Healing Power* is a timely and informative book offering practical techniques for blending shamanic healing practices with traditional medicine to maximize the body's innate healing energy and take one's power back to create shifts in health."

— **Bryn Blankinship, CMHt, CI,** The Regression Specialist,© certified hypnotherapist, and author of *The Limitless Soul*

"With deep commitment and passion Dr. Martin offers us a bridge to merge Western medicine with shamanic and energy healing, giving us new tools and perspective with our health and lives. She asks that we activate our consciousness and awareness (and connection to Spirit, God, Nature) and suggests that through this we can affect our health and our lives. She offers great questions and tools, which can take us beyond the old beliefs that limit our expression and our health and also opens us to possibilities we may not have yet seen."

— **Lynn Berryhill,** artist, energy medicine practitioner, and senior faculty at the Four Winds Society

"This is a book the world needs for understanding complete healing. I especially recommend this guide for people in the medical or healing fields who want to deepen their communication and their understanding of clients' needs, in a very organized fashion. This book has real tools that can be used with every single client with tangible ways for every level of healing needed. If you want to 'just' deepen the connection with your client, this is the book for you. This guide can revolutionize the medical world."

— **Georgia Herrera, D.C.,** owner of Sacred Mother Healing Center and host of *Sacred Magic* Radio

"Dr. Sharon Martin gives us the keys to healing from around the world. Learn about exceptional techniques and principles—the ancient and the new, the technical and the intuitive, the medical and the mystical, and the tribal and the traditional. They are all here for us to discover and to use. Most importantly, Dr. Martin introduces us to our own innermost healer, awakening the sublime shaman within us all!"

— **Sharon Anne Klingler,** medium, spiritualist minister, and author of *Answers from the Ancestral Realms* and *Power Words*

This book is dedicated to my father, Gordon Anthony Martin,
who first admonished me when I was starting medical school
"Physician, heal thyself!"

He went on to tell me there was more to healing than prescriptions
and that I needed to teach people about the other ways. He said,
"Sharon, you need to write a book."

Dad, here it is, 30 years later, just as you wanted.

Contents

Foreword by *Carl Greer, Ph.D., Psy.D.*   9

Preface   12

○

PART ONE
Understanding Maximum Medicine

1   Walk with Me   16

2   Evolution of a Healer   25

3   Why Western Medicine Is Not Enough   35

○

PART TWO
Maximum Medicine Fundamentals

4   Bring Back the Mystical   52

5   Layer upon Layer, the Power Builds: The Chacana and the
Medicine Wheels   63

6   The Medicine Wheels of Inner Actions and Inner Tasks   82

7   Consciousness, Character, and Connecting to Spirit   95

8   Lose the Story, Lose the Past   109

◆
PART THREE
Applying Maximum Medicine through the Four 'A's

9   Maximum Medicine: Become Aware   118

10   Allow   135

11   Act with Intention   154

12   Affirm with Ritual   164

13   The Maximum Medicine Approach to Common
     Health Challenges   181

     Afterword   191

     Medicine Wheels and Chacana   192

     Notes   196

     Bibliography   199

     Resources   202

     Index   204

     Acknowledgments   206

     About the Author   207

Foreword

Western medicine has made great strides over the years in surgical and pharmaceutical treatments, but despite this progress, when it comes to mortality rates, chronic diseases, conditions such as diabetes, and mental illness, the US does not compare well to other countries. What's more, our health care costs are higher per capita than in most other places, and many of our citizens lack even the most basic health care. As the for-profit sector buys up medical practices and hospitals, individual doctors face the pressure of seeing ever more patients and spending less time with them. They recognize that the undisputed value of the doctor–patient relationship is being diminished.

Day to day, Dr. Martin works under the pressures of the US healthcare system, so she well understands the challenges. Fortunately, she has found ways to help patients have greater control over their health. The practices she offers in *Maximize Your Healing Power: Shamanic Healing Techniques to Overcome Your Health Challenges* can be used to empower patients as well as make doctors more effective in their work.

Dr. Martin earned a Ph.D. in Physiology, worked and taught in the Department of Medicine at Emory University, served as a department chief at a hospital, and now works in a rural medicine clinic in Pennsylvania. She is a rare blend of an accomplished academic researcher and compassionate, practical healer, who incorporates into her patient care, teachings from shamanism and various energy medicine traditions. Her dedication to studying these important healing modalities is evident in her clear explanations of why the practices she recommends can make a difference for patients seeking better health.

Because of her training in non-Western healing methods, Dr. Martin recognizes that the universal energy of Source is found in its component energies—the elements, power animals, ascended masters, and so forth. She describes how we can learn to call forth and work with these various energies, using inner-work practices she teaches her patients so they can access inner wisdom and energy to effectuate healing. Thus Dr. Martin empowers her patients to take an active part in their recovery.

"Healing" comes from the word "whole," and to become healed in a holistic sense requires approaches that not only get one back to their homeostasis before their illness but, ideally, back to an even healthier homeostasis or way of being. Recognizing this holistic way of looking at health and wellness, Dr. Martin skillfully explores mind–body–spirit connections and how people with no training in energy medicine can work with powerful practices that can help them achieve outcomes they otherwise might have felt were unattainable.

Many in the mind–body–spirit wellness field talk about how shamanic and energy medicine practices can be beneficial, but Dr. Martin goes a step further and stresses the importance of bringing their gains into everyday life. She shows how they can be used to support patients in being more diligent in taking their medicine and making lifestyle changes in the realms of exercise, nutrition, and stress management, leading to clear health improvements.

Dr. Martin also writes about the importance of how we relate to our health and any health conditions we might have. Facts are facts. What we do with them can vary. For example, a seemingly unmovable thought such as *I have high blood pressure just like my father, and there's nothing I can do about it besides take medicine* might not be so unmovable after all.

Dr. Martin explains that by connecting with Source, the creative energy of the universe, we can develop a wider viewpoint and become less restrictive in our thinking. What's more, we can learn to interact with unseen realms and the wisdom and energy we find there that can affect our bodies, minds, and emotions.

By using her practices, readers will find even that the most frightening diagnoses do not have to devastate them. For example, a diagnosis of aggressive cancer can understandably trigger a reaction of despair and the belief that, "My life is over. There's nothing I can do but prepare to die." However, it can also elicit a response of hopeful curiosity about what one can do to treat the disease and maybe even become free of it. The latter can lead to reflection on the questions of "Why now?" and "How does my developing aggressive cancer figure into my life going forward?" and "What do I want to do in the time I have left? What 'I love you's' and 'Please forgive me's' and 'I forgive you's' do I need to say?" A difficult diagnosis might lead to the question, "What energetic approaches can I engage in to achieve healing, even if I don't survive?" and a willingness to work often with the practices presented in this book. Healing might mean coming to a place where one can say, "I am at peace with the life I have lived" and "I am accepting of whatever comes next," an attitude that might even prolong life.

People with a variety of health concerns will benefit from Dr. Martin's sage advice and practical approach to maximizing one's natural ability to bring about healing. Her Book *Maximize Your Healing Power* makes a significant contribution to the field of self-healing and fills in some of the gaps that Western medicine alone is often not able to address.

— **Carl Greer, Ph.D., Psy.D.,** psychotherapist and author of
Change Your Story, Change Your Life and
Change the Story of Your Health

Preface

I love scientific facts. I love certainty. Over the years, when I have had cause to reflect on where I sit on the far edge of the spontaneity curve (at the end of not-so-spontaneous), I think back to my childhood, which was one of unpredictability and chaos, one in which I lacked control, and I can rationalize why I came to love science and medicine.

In these fields, black is black, and white is white. The Latin name for a tendon will always be the same. An enzyme pathway has components that are set and known. The knee bone is always connected to the hip bone. One can draw a mental picture of a client using cellular structure and biochemistry and feel certain that the disease process is just so, and that the choice of therapeutics (decided by how they fit with the science of the disease) always will lead to healing. Or will it?

During my years as a physician trained in Internal Medicine with a background as researcher and teacher of physiology, I respected the science behind diagnoses and expected to be able to effect direct healing in my patients. But niggling contradictions and unexpected effects of stand-ard protocols kept appearing: a lab test that carried me down a pathway toward an expected diagnosis somehow ended elsewhere; the patients' body chemistries did not follow the "textbook" recovery plan.

Our medical treatments do not always engage the patient or create a beneficial psychosocial environment for healing. How can we expect healing when, on the one hand, the prescription is working well, but on the other, it costs the patient $400 out of pocket each month? We may improve the patient's chemistry but worsen their health and well-being when we ignore their emotional and spiritual aspects. The belief that heal-ing physical ailments is black and white does not account for the fluidity of the human condition, does not speak to the miraculous, and does not honor the alchemy of unpredictable outcomes.

As I waded into the zones of gray and saw their ubiquity, my eyes opened to what I have come to believe as a core truth: We humans are more than science has described; we have immense power in controlling our personal and collective destinies; and we are surrounded by forces greater than ourselves and can ally ourselves with these forces for our betterment.

These observations form the premise behind this book. My fervent wish is for you, the reader, to feel empowered when it comes to your health and wellness and to know that you have control over your life.

In *Maximize Your Healing Power: Shamanic Healing Techniques to Overcome Your Health Challenges*, I will show you how I think about the bigger picture of wellness so that you can start feeling your way into the magnificent mysteries that affect you. I will teach you ways you can expand your view of yourself, amplifying the power of the positive choices you make on a day-to-day basis and improving your healing journey's outcome. My teachings are constructed within the frameworks of shamanism and energy medicine because my life has been illuminated, enhanced, and expanded by these concepts and techniques, and I believe you can experience the same.

In this book, I share what I see as a gaping divide between Western medicine and indigenous shamanic and energy techniques and then show you how I learned to see the bigger picture of medicine by looking through a lens of science combined with shamanism. I offer stories and step-by-step practices and techniques you can use. If you really dig in and engage with these practices with discipline and commitment, such as doing the meditations/journeys and keeping a journal of your insights and progress, you will know what it is to have heightened awareness and power and gain new perspectives and you will be bridging the healing gap and enjoying greater vitality and life force.

This is my heartfelt wish for you.

Note: the patient and client examples in this book are altered so as to not identify the person; they are often composites of patient encounters.

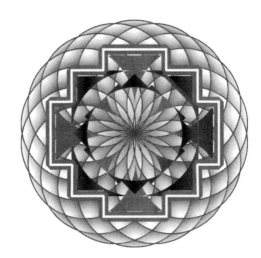

Part One

UNDERSTANDING
MAXIMUM
MEDICINE

1

Walk with Me

My tipping point toward learning about shamanic practice and energy medicine came completely unexpectedly. I opened a clinic in rural Pennsylvania about 18 years ago and was faced every day with the differences between Western medicine and what felt to me like a more holistic healing approach.

One day, a Friday evening, about 5 o'clock, after a long week of seeing patients back to back, I was exhausted and ready to drop. The drive home was about 30 miles, and I was eager to get started. I came out of the exam room and stood at the counter in the nurses' station to finish up my paperwork for the last patient. I looked up and saw the receptionist walking down the hall from the main lobby, a worried look on her face. She told me a young man had come into the office with his girlfriend—he was not our patient—complaining of anxiety and looking agitated. The receptionist had talked over the situation with one of the nurses; they both thought it was important that I see this patient.

My mind was a tumble of thoughts, some of them not so charitable because of the time and possible needs. Doesn't he have his own doctor (meaning, why do I have to work late on a Friday night)? What if he is clinically psychiatric (meaning, how am I going to get the state police or ambulance here to bring him to a psychiatric facility; or, what if it takes the police two hours to get here and I am stuck waiting)? Do we have to restrain him if he needs psychiatric admission and refuses to go (am I putting my staff in an unsafe position)?

I took the young man into the exam room while his girlfriend sat in the waiting room. Something told me to put away the computer and paper; I turned my gaze to him and just sat. He was handsome and youthful, with soft blonde hair that curled gently on his head. Later, I reflected that he looked like a cherub. He began to tell me of the vivid dreams he had every night; dreams about things that would happen to people he knew and sometimes to people he had never met. Mostly, the dreams were about bad outcomes for the people that showed up in them. In the daytime, he could not get the images out of his head. The worry was disrupting his sleep and his ability to find peace.

The key thing in psychiatry, at least at the level of a general practitioner, is whether these images are hallucinations or whether his beliefs were paranoid or delusional. Was he simply having a bipolar episode with his mind racing and his problems sleeping and eating? I decided to call his girlfriend back to the exam room. When he has these dreams, I asked her, do they come true? Do they yield accurate predictions? Yes, she said. Then I asked whether anyone else had noticed his ability to predict the future. Again, her answer was yes. In fact, his grandmother was a Romani and told the family when this young man was a toddler that he had "the sight."

The more I learned about him, the more I realized that Western medicine's approach would not be helpful and might even be harmful. First, he was not crazy, and no amount of medication would fix what was ailing him. He had heightened intuitive skills, even predictive skills. The most psychiatry could offer was antianxiety medications, which would be sedating at best. And pushing this lovely young man into the medical system would cause him to be labeled as defective or "cracked," which he was not. Rather, he was extremely intuitive and empathic—traits that are undervalued in our society. What he really needed to learn was when to allow his "seeing" to occur, to make it on his terms. In a sense, he needed to gain mastery over his perceptions.

I told him how I saw his issues and that I did not think he was crazy. That was all he wanted to know. The relief on his face when I said this was reassuring to him and rewarding to me. Had I not seen this issue from an out-of-the-box perspective, things would have turned out a lot differently. I suggested that he seek out some renowned intuitives and find out how they learned to master their "sight." He left the office that day calmer and reassured. I left the office committed to learning a new way of "seeing" things myself.

Not long after, I began in-depth shamanic energy training with Alberto Villoldo, Ph.D., founder of the Four Winds Society, an organization that teaches healing of the luminous energy body. Over the last, nearly 20 years, I have studied with some master healers, some of whom are very intuitive as they work with the energy body, while some follow techniques passed down from the elders of indigenous cultures. The commonality among all my teachers is that they firmly believe the pathways to health and well-being are much broader and deeper than those used in Western medicine. I have come to agree with them.

I have watched and heard from patients over the years about their distress with the system of medicine in the United States. (I think the challenges in neighboring Canada, for example, are likely different. There, cost is taken out of the equation, although perhaps patients must wait longer to get in to see a specialist.) Here is an example of what patients might go through when they come to the office for a medical appointment in the United States.

The office feels industrial. Your copay is $15 more than it was last year, or your deductible is huge. Your appointment is for 10:00 and it's already 10:30. You had to take time off work to come to the appointment—every hour you miss work is more money out of your pocket. You have belly pain and occasional diarrhea, and you are scared you have colon cancer. Somewhere in your family tree is someone who had colon cancer, and you wonder whether you are cursed with that genetic predisposition. You haven't seen any blood in your stool, but you have read that sometimes colon cancer can happen without any blood. Meanwhile, you have your mask on because you're scared to death to be in a medical facility when deadly respiratory diseases are circulating in the community.

When you finally get to the exam room, you are asked to put on a paper-thin gown for examination and are freezing and one step shy of a full-blown panic attack. Should you sit on the exam table, which is uncomfortable, or in the chair? How much longer is the doctor going to be? Do they disinfect the exam tables between patients?

The doctor arrives, wearing a mask, and hardly looks at you; she just types on her laptop. You tell her you have diarrhea sometimes and your belly hurts. You ask whether you could have colon cancer? She says, "Oh, you just have irritable bowel. You need more fiber." She goes on to say you are on the young side for colon cancer, and you do not have a high-risk family history, but she will have you do stool cards to look for hidden blood. Meanwhile, start taking Metamucil each night and cut out all soda and artificial sweeteners.

Your mind is spinning. You do not drink soda and don't use artificial sweeteners. Why didn't she just ask you? How is Metamucil going to help? You are already almost vegan in your diet and eat lots of plant-based foods. Why do you need more fiber? The doctor leaves the room having never asked about your belly pain.

You have a moment of real self-reflection, as the question you want to be asked by your doctor is now foremost in your brain: When did this all start? You remember back to three months ago, when you broke up with your lousy boyfriend after you caught him cheating on you, and you argued, and he said you were never a good lover. Tears come to your eyes. Why didn't she have more time to talk about what is really going on inside you? What is going on will not be fixed by Metamucil, of that you are certain. You are starting to get angry, and you are still freezing cold as you sit there in a hospital gown. You are still scared and sad, and you still have not received any help.

Nothing is worse than feeling under the control of a system that is terribly broken. This example could be replaced by any symptom, any office visit, and the complaints would still be the same: Too much money, too little personal time, you don't feel heard or listened to, you're confused about what to do to take care of yourself, and you're angry that you have to leave your health in the hands of this broken mess.

The concerns about not having enough time and not being listened to are present in the Canadian and UK health systems as well as here in the United States. Even if you are very proactive about your well-being, you would like information to guide you on what you can do for yourself; you have questions and would like some answers.

I, myself, am fed up with the state of today's Western medicine. I am a board-certified, internal medicine physician who works at a clinic in rural south-central Pennsylvania. I know how to do "standard of care" academic medicine, how to diagnose disease, how to choose appropriate treatment, and how to get the numbers of your lab results back to the "healthy" range. However, I am increasingly dissatisfied having to push a volume of patients through just to pay the bills. I do not like having to click certain boxes in the computer just to make the documentation requirements for the insurance companies. I want to sit, talk, guide, and teach you. I want to have conversations that help you make healthy choices and nudge you toward taking better care of yourself.

I wrote this book to help you back into the driver's seat of your health and well-being. In addition to being a Western-trained physician, I am also a shamanic practitioner who heals through the luminous energy field. In other words, I am also an energy practitioner.

Through my training with Dr. Alberto Villoldo and the Four Winds Society, I learned that The Luminous Energy Field (LEF)—also called the *light body, halo,* or *aura*—is a matrix that envelops and informs the physical structure of all living beings and organizes the body in the same way that iron filings are organized by a magnet. It is a reservoir of vital force—a sea of living energy as indispensable to our health as the oxygen and nutrients carried by the bloodstream. These energies are the purest and most precious fuel for life. When the vital reserves are depleted through illness, environmental pollutants, or stress, we suffer disease.[1]

This book is a compilation of processes and techniques that, I believe, will teach you how to heal by adopting a different perspective. I will show you how you can blend the Western approach your doctor prescribes for you with powerful practices and awarenesses gleaned from the indigenous ways of healing. You will be shown step-by-step ways to learn about your energy field, to increase your awareness and control over your field, to not only shift the trajectory of a health challenge but also to amplify your immune system and well-being. Even in the absence of a health challenge, you can use this book to increase your ability to thrive in your world, increasingly empowered.

As you work with this book, you will be shown how to see your health from different perspectives. I will teach you how to increase awareness— of your body, of your energy field, of the world around you. You will learn how to sense forces and energies of the unseen world. These forces influence our health by impacting our energy body, so awareness is the first step toward mitigating the impact. In common with our indigenous ancestors, you will become more deeply connected to Nature, which, in and of itself, amplifies your personal power. Your intuition will expand, and you will gain mastery over your intention and your own energy field— characteristics that are vital to self-healing. These abilities are valuable not just innately but also when used in concert with and as a complement to the brilliant technologies of Western medicine.

Some of the practices in this book are rituals; most have a spiritual quality. By this I mean that inherent to all these practices is the philosophical belief that we humans are not alone in the Universe; that we are not separate from Nature, from the Divine, from the Cosmos. Thus, when we heal through and within the luminous field, we are engaging aspects of ourselves that are integrally linked to the universal matrix, giving us access to power and forces greater than us.

Each process or practice I teach is valuable inherently, even as a stand-alone process. You can work with each one specifically and after gaining familiarity and mastery, you will find yourself feeling more enlivened. For example, I will show you several ways to enhance your intuition. Even if you do not apply this learning to your health, being more intuitive will serve you well in life—to sense when to have more caution, when to step in and act, when to be more of an observer. The techniques I teach in this book will help you to expand your perspective—from looking at the literal, to experiencing the emotional, to standing back as the observer watching your soul's journey. You will take in data in a new way and have a better command over your energy field and thus be more able to steer your life in the direction you choose.

As you apply these abilities to your energy body, you gain downstream beneficial effects in your physical health. For example, imagine you are having a stressful day at work and your belly is grumbling and cramping. You will be aware that there might be a connection and will know how to stop for a moment, move your consciousness into communication with Nature or the Divine, and with the eyes of an impartial observer, see daily stress whirling around you. You will see those energies as separate from you. This awareness allows you to move yourself out of the currents of pain and unease and back into sync with the reservoir of life force. Also, you now will reflect on what things changed in your diet that have impacted how you feel, or what interactions you had, whether they went badly, and how you might change them in the future so they do not contribute to ill health. The greater the amount of knowledge you gain, the greater the amount of control you accumulate over your energy body, which influences your physical health. You will learn that you are no longer buffeted about by life but now are more able to choose the direction of your path.

Many patients over the years have shown me that when they feel able to make conscious choices and feel more in control of the energy affecting their health, their resilience and potential for self-healing increases.

A patient I'll call Pete has been a type I diabetic since his teens. This means that he is dependent on taking the hormone insulin—without it, he would die. He injected his insulin daily but had not adjusted the doses based on his blood sugar readings, and as a result, his overall sugar level was too high. Uncontrolled sugars are known to add to plaque buildup in the blood vessels. Pete had coronary artery disease in his late 40s and had already undergone cardiac bypass surgery.

If that wasn't a big enough burden to carry, Pete had low blood sugars, especially when he hiked mountain ridges during hunting season. To have a low blood sugar level is a frightening event and is life threatening. I asked Pete repeatedly to consider getting an insulin pump, a machine that measures blood sugars moment by moment and delivers small amounts of insulin in response. Diabetics with insulin pumps have much better control of their blood sugar and avoid low sugars. For years, Pete declined.

One year, I tried a different tack other than the usual "We need your sugars better controlled so you don't get kidney disease or lose your vision." I made a change informed by my shamanic training. I shifted my perspective out of the literal scientific approach into the personalized. I asked him, "Is this the best your life can be?" I spoke to him from the level of his life journey. I asked him how it felt to have his hiking limited by the fear of a low sugar. I asked him if he was scared alone on the mountainside when his sugar dropped. And I said, "Are there things we can do to help avoid those moments?"

Five months later, at his routine appointment, Pete told me he was ready for an insulin pump—six years after I had been hounding him! Since then, he has had no low sugars and hikes easily without fear! I shifted *my* perspective, and *his* life (and mine) changed. You too will learn how to make shifts in perspective and then watch how your life changes.

Even if you have never done shamanic or energy medicine work before, I will help you get started and encourage you to develop your self-healing abilities. In the resources section at the end of this book, you'll find lists of groups and practitioners I trust to help you do shamanic healing work. They might be able to help you do more effective, powerful work than you could do on your own initially, and I would trust any of them with my own health.

As a physician who does shamanic healing work, I am not immune to the stressors we all face that challenge our health and well-being. For many of us, the year 2020 was a year that presented the biggest test to our wellness we had ever encountered: COVID-19. We had to deal with the possibility of catching a virus with unknown consequences for ourselves, recognizing that even people who seemed to be younger and healthier than us were dying from this virulent disease. On top of that, our brains and psyches were strained with the overlay of the media reports, changing information and guidance, alternative theories, and the huge amount of scary possibilities associated with COVID.

I admit that each day at work I struggled with apprehension and sometimes outright fear. I had to dig in to find reserves of resilience and equanimity. I was especially challenged, coming close to blowing a gasket, whenever someone walked into the office mask-less past two swinging doors that clearly said, "Masks required," past elderly infirm people sitting in the waiting room. Always by my side were my go-to helpers: spirit guides, sacred space, Nature, meditations, and energy-clearing techniques. (I teach you about all of these later in the book.) I likely would have gone under mentally had I not had these foundations to turn to. My immunity feels stable as I turn again and again to my shamanic teachings and practices.

A Shamanic Perspective

My teachings come with some assumptions, some cosmology that you do not have to ascribe to but should know about as you are learning. I first learned about shamanism in the Healing the Light Body school. My teacher, Alberto Villoldo, has translated the cosmology of the Q'ero Indians of Peru. The stories of the luminous field and how Inca shamans worked within the universal energy field, which we are all woven into, are admittedly spun with Western language and viewpoints. What I learned is several generations away and culturally distant from the original. What I teach comes also from other mystics; this book shares an eclectic mix of wisdom teachings.

I believe there is a universal matrix of energy that we are all a part of, and that we contribute to, and that has divine intelligence. I believe that healing done at the level of the personal energy body is powerful, long lasting, and accesses the source of physiologic illness. I believe we have a soul and that our souls communicate with Spirit. I believe in reincarnation. I believe that the life force and its intelligence permeate everything on Earth and in the galaxy.

According to a professor of psychology at Seattle University, Kevin Krycka, Ph.D.:

> Shamanism is defined as a system of spiritual healing with methods designed to promote the well-being of mind, body, and soul . . . [it] defines the shaman as a technician, in this case as a spiritual healer–technician, who performs rituals (e.g., journey and soul retrieval) intended to create sacred space wherein healing can take place.[2]

I agree that my goal as a shamanic practitioner, energy practitioner, and your teacher is to show you methods designed to promote well-being across the entire human spectrum—mind, body, spirit, and soul.

We Westerners who call ourselves shamans or "shamanic practitioners" have incorporated much from the indigenous: belief in the power of the natural world and its inhabitants, use of trance (deep meditation or visualization) to gain knowledge, use of rituals to set up a request to Spirit for intervention, and belief that we are connected to Earth and the galaxy. Indigenous shamans saw a very thin line, or even no line, between physical, emotional, and spiritual health. If you study shamanism, whether you learn from Aboriginal healers, Tlingit throat singers, Hopi elders, Laika of the Andes, or others, what is most important to me is for you to develop links to the unseen world, to see yourself as part of the universal matrix, and be able to have increased control over your luminous energy field, which in turn gives you control over your holistic health.

With the viewpoints and processes I teach in this book, you will have the ability to shift the course of your health. If you are not physically challenged but seek greater vitality and confidence, these shamanic techniques and practices are highly effective. Step into the power of self-awareness as you learn how to be in charge of your energy structure and your physiology, both of which the luminous field shaped and continually influenced. At the very least, learn and incorporate these teachings so that the next time you must go to a doctor's appointment, you can proceed with authority over your health, knowing more of what you want to obtain from the visit, and energized to make that happen. Come. Walk with me.

Evolution of a Healer

I never knew that I would be a physician. My path to becoming one was steered by events I did not plan, at least not in a conscious way. I always loved science, loved nature, loved understanding things about the world—rocks, plants, birds. I wanted to be a veterinarian.

When I was in high school, my family lived in Thailand, where my father worked for the United States Department of State as an expert on China. I had it all figured out—I had a dream one night of farmland and a silo. Sitting looking at a map one day I thought about Kansas, so I researched veterinary school in Kansas. Excitedly, I wrote for an application, and as I remember, I started filling it out. Then my father got wind of my plan, and, well, suffice to say, "Dorothy, you are not in Kansas!"

My dad was a strong personality, with definite opinions that left little room for negotiation. Because my immediate family would still be living overseas when I started college, he refused to let me live in a location so far removed from any relatives. My grandparents lived in Connecticut, so I changed my applications to schools in the Northeast. I got accepted to an Ivy League school, but again my father's decisions reigned. I had to accept admission to a school that offered me financial aid, so I started college in a town near my grandparents. Almost as soon as I started, I was miserable.

By this time, my mother and siblings had moved back to the Washington, DC, area, and my father went back overseas to Southeast Asia to work. I moved back home, which was now in Maryland, to finish my last year of college and then started looking for work that I thought would give me a good scientific background to apply to vet school. My path got steered again, by things I never saw coming.

I was working a menial job in the science field at the National Institutes of Health, when I met a scientist from the graduate school across the street (Uniformed Services University of the Health Sciences) and, out of the blue, he asked me if I wanted to go to graduate school and get a doctorate in physiology.

I love physiology—how the cells of different organs perform such different tasks, and how everything works in such a smooth, miraculous way. The first time I saw the waves drawn out on paper while recording an electrocardiogram, I was moved and inspired. I had not yet been accepted to vet school, and when I learned that being a graduate student at the Uniformed Services University did not require joining the military, and that there was no tuition and studying there paid a stipend that was more than I was making, well, no brainer!

After graduate school, I stumbled across the country to California, following a romantic partner, only to have our relationship fall apart when I arrived. The next 18 months were a blur of depression and unhappiness. Desperate, I called an old boss from my National Institutes of Health days who was now a professor in Atlanta and begged for a job to get me as far away from California as I could, back closer to home on the East Coast. Miraculously, he had a job for me, so I moved to Atlanta, where I worked as a researcher and teacher in the Department of Medicine at Emory University.

I was still depressed, so I was fortunate to get help from an amazing psychiatrist whom I was seeing in therapy. In our sessions, he never told me what to do, and in fact, almost never spoke and let me come to all my own conclusions. One day during our session, I was grumbling about my job as a research scientist.

"Writing grants is a thankless job," I complained. "You can be a brilliant mind with spectacular writing, and your grant likely won't get funded. The odds are against you because grant money is limited."

"I want you to apply to medical school," my psychiatrist blurted out.

I was shocked. His directive was so out of character that it gave me pause. He rarely said anything, much less give me a directive. He did not elaborate, but just hearing his voice with strong instruction made me take notice.

I had a lot of apprehension about applying to medical school because I was afraid of anatomy class—the volume of material you must memorize, material with Latin names difficult even to pronounce—and there were abundant stories of how difficult school would be. But knowing my psychiatrist believed in me enough to step out of character and instruct me made me feel that going to medical school and earning a degree was possible for me. So, despite being apprehensive, I did apply and did get accepted.

When I look back on this moment, I see divine providence at work. Over the years, I have come to see more clearly a spiritual overlay to everything I do, and I believe that it is the same for all humans. I learned about the energy field that surrounds each living creature and is integrated into the universal energy field (this idea is taught in energy medicine and most forms of shamanism) and how it has a deeply spiritual nature. Also, because I have had many exposures to the paranormal and insights into the unseen world, sensing a greater intelligence permeating the path I walked did not feel unusual to me.

As a kid, I often had moments of "woo-woo" similar to those that many people have experienced. I would know who was calling when the phone rang. I would dream of something, and a few days later, that something would occur. My sister and I loved to explore the metaphysical world. We read stories of Edgar Cayce, books by Jane Roberts who channeled SETH, and the Carlos Castaneda books on Don Juan, a Mexican seer. We would travel to downtown Washington, DC, to visit a woman psychic who did tarot readings; she told us things about our lives at the current time and into the future. On the way home, my sister and I would talk about how facts of our lives could be known by a stranger. We decided that surely that meant that destiny or some sort of divine intelligence had a prominent hand in determining our paths.

When I look back on the crooked path I walked to become a physician, I can see serendipitous moments when I was influenced to step a particular direction—more evidence to me that divine instruction is in play.

Another serendipitous moment came when I first picked up my copy of Alberto Villoldo's book *Shaman, Healer, Sage*. I had come across this book by chance, felt drawn to it, and begun reading. For whatever reason, as I looked at the photo on the cover of Alberto's face with a picture of Machu Picchu behind him, a buzz and tingle came over me. Having experienced wild moments before, I was not completely surprised by my sense of being nudged toward shamanism. Luckily, I paid attention to that buzz, and signed up for the author's Healing the Light Body School training program at The Four Winds Society.

Over the subsequent years studying shamanic energy techniques, I came to learn the importance of those quiet signals, either in my body or around me. Messages come to us from all directions. A whisper in your ear, a grabbing in your gut, the way the blue jay on the back deck seems to catch your eye, how the woods go quiet when you reach a certain point on the trail—knowledge can be gained in many situations. As you will learn, to gain knowledge from the greater world around you, you will have to heighten your awareness, be receptive to information that comes to you intuitively, and be ready to use that information in ways you may not have used before. I will teach you ways to accomplish these things.

One of the biggest points of education for me came with my understanding of what it means to be a healer. This understanding did not happen all at once but was learned piece by piece after experiencing events in Western medicine that could certainly have gone better.

My Eyes Are Opened

I was in medical school when I got my first glimpse of a place where Western medicine can fall short. In their third year, students start their clinical rotations. Each month, we were assigned to a different specialty— Medicine, Psychiatry, Surgery, Pediatrics, and so on. Because we knew next to nothing, we formed the rear of our work group. In front were the leaders: the attending physician and the assistant chief of service (a resident who was staying on an extra year to be in a teaching capacity), who were known by their knee-length white coats. Behind them were the medical residents (already graduated from medical school and now training in their specialty). They also had long coats, and these were often rumpled and scruffy because the residents were chronically exhausted. Medical students were identified by their short white jackets. I quickly learned the hierarchy of coat length: medical students had the least coat and the least authority.

Down the halls of the hospital we would go, like ducklings, entering each patient's room, one by one. The group would stand at the foot of each patient's bed; usually the room was so small that the group of eight or so would spill out into the hall. The attending physician then would grill the residents on medical facts about each case.

One morning, we stopped into the room of an elderly patient who was admitted to the hospital for a life-threatening abnormality in her heart's electrical cadence (arrhythmia). The attending physician sought to make teaching points by telling the group the statistics and prognosis for this condition. As we gathered at the patient's bedside, we were led on a discussion of the patient's likelihood of dying from the arrhythmia. Here we were, a group of white-coated strangers, standing at the bedside, talking literally in the air above the patient, and figuratively above her under-standing of details, about how close she was to death.

I was horrified and angry, perhaps more so than some of my fellow students. After all, I was the eldest member of our medical class and had lived a life outside medical school, and thus, was less likely to blindly trust authority or take anyone's word as gospel.

I felt that the physician should have stopped long enough to say, "Hello, Mrs. So-and-So. How are you feeling today? We are going to talk about the science behind your disease, and please chime in. We'll be talk-ing about numbers like the probabilities with this diagnosis, but those won't necessarily apply to you." Instead, he was cold and analytical. Where was the compassion? We did nothing to make her feel better; I think that we did harm.

Another day, we had a patient with a lung disease. She was clearly vulnerable, and my fellow medical student, despite knowing how pain-ful it can be to have a needle pushed into your wrist to take an arterial blood sample if it is not done exactly right, jabbed her again and again as I steadied the woman's wrist. We had been taught that you should stop after three pokes and call an expert, and here she was trying a fourth time. Seeing the patient wince and grit her teeth, I said something like, "Do you want to call someone?" but my fellow student ignored me and bulldozed ahead. As I recall, she got it in on the ninth try. I still feel badly about not being more assertive, but at the time, I didn't want to say too much in front of the patient and have her lose confidence in our team.

I did not stand up to the culture in those particular situations as a med-ical student, but later, when I was in class with the physician and professor who had been so insensitive when discussing a patient's condition in front of her, I questioned his approach often. I was an A student in my other classes, but he gave me a D. I learned my lesson: Do not go up against an authority figure in the field of medicine.

In medical school, I did not put a lot of thought into what it meant to be a healer; I just knew that I did not like how those experiences felt. It pushed me to choose a residency in a community hospital instead of an Ivy League academic center, because I felt a community-based hospital might not have such a strong culture of one-upmanship. I wanted to be in a more relaxed environment, where doctors would learn from each other as they talked about treating patients with compassion. Later, I would start a clinic in a rural area in south-central Pennsylvania, where I work today, guided by the belief that the patient is a partner in healing who should always be treated with respect and compassion.

Over the years, I have always tried to connect with patients personally before launching into the medical conversation, making eye contact and using their name. If they have a life-threatening condition, I don't immediately launch into the medical explanation. I explain how much danger they're in using layman's terms, saying, "There are risks in what is happening, but here is what we are going to do to lessen those risks." I would never treat a patient the way I saw some physicians treating them when I was a student.

Now, I want to be clear that I am not telling you this story to make me seem special or amazing or unique at all, but rather, to share my attempts at being a compassionate human within my Western medical training. Sometimes, it has been a challenge, but I do my best anyway.

Two Patients Seek Healing

I treated two women in my medical practice who both had had recent diagnoses of cancer. One woman (I'll call her Jane) was plagued with worry and wanted her blood work tested more often than is traditionally called for. She cried much of the time while I was treating her and seemed fixated on the disease and how it might conquer her. Jane was miserable although she was undergoing treatment and her cancer was in remission. She could not seem to step outside her diagnosis: She was caged by her fear. Because of my shamanic training, I was able to sense that her energy field was constricted and dense. Her vitality was significantly diminished. Despite my attempts to encourage her to shift her perspective, she kept reliving and ruminating over the moment she was diagnosed. Jane's view of her world was directed by her fears, which ran rampant inside her mind, keeping her stuck in anxiety-provoking thought processes. She was stuck and could not see the possibility of any path except one laden by fear that moved quickly toward death.

The second patient (I will call her Jill), who also had cancer but at a slightly worse stage, started off her discussions with me about what she could do to improve her immunity and health while she was getting chemotherapy and radiation therapy. Jill adopted a healthier diet, began a walking program, and kept a journal of all the things she loves in the world. She has shifted her focus away from her diagnosis and out to the world, noticing the sunrise, giving thanks for the beauty of the wood-pecker that frequents her bird feeder.

Who is cured? Neither—at least, not yet. However, I know that Jill has set the stage for a more optimal outcome for healing, not necessarily her body (she may not experience that) but her spirit. Jill seems to be healing from her fear, from her powerlessness, and learning to accept uncertainty and take charge of her thoughts and perspectives.

Let me explain.

I have come to see healing as experiential. You do not have to change anything in your physical body to have an experience of healing. The walk toward healing involves either a sense of reinterpreting what you are experiencing in the literal world or a shift in your energy field brought about by rituals and practices I teach in this book. The shift in your energy field then informs your experience.

Healing involves having a greater acceptance and willingness to continue engaging life with optimism. Someone who feels ill or broken or wounded or defective can feel as if she is caught in a box with no air holes, unable to see a future because her view of something grander is constrained. Two of the keys in the shamanic practices I learned (and teach) are to shift perspective and to exercise your ability to sense the forces from the unseen world connected to you and operating in alliance with you.

Healing, as I define it, comes when you make peace with where your soul is on your life's path, holding a renewed excitement about extending your human journey or a willingness to move forward and even experience a sense of renewal. You may not be able to fully heal from a physical ailment or disease, but you can still experience healing.

I have come to see many people struggling with health challenges as being locked in a box of their diagnosis. Many patients I care for have debilitating back pain. Several are under 40 years of age and define their lives based on this diagnosis. Each time they come to the office, their main goal is directed at getting narcotics for their pain. They are stuck, as if blocked in concrete, self-identified as disabled, and often unwilling to consider any approach other than narcotics to given them some relief. To me, healing them means helping them break open their box to show them there's life outside of their limited diagnosis, outside of being stuck.

When you are healed, you are not stuck. Your physicality may not have changed but you are not stuck. You are willing and able to see something different as a treatment and something different as an outcome. Maybe that means going to acupuncture, maybe getting an MRI, and finding an anesthesiologist who can give you an epidural. The willingness to broaden your perspective pokes air holes in your box.

Healing Stage 4 cancer might involve reflecting on your life and recognizing a unique opportunity to teach others, such as your family—using ideas such as "I can spread love while I'm still here, be sure I'm the one that brings the flowers to church on Sunday, lead the lay prayer"—because you are not stuck ruminating about your death sentence.

Healing is about being receptive to other possibilities about what you can experience and how you can heal—and being open to staying as vital as possible.

In the practices I teach in this book, you will learn to sense your energy body, gain a deeper awareness of your physical body, improve your intuition to get messages about how to proceed, and sense forces and intelligences outside yourself that can be harnessed for guidance and power. In shifting perspective and energy, you can take charge of your health and life experience and become more fully immersed and participative in life. If you choose to work with a healer (including your physician), this work will be in partnership.

You do not have to have a health challenge to gain from the teachings in this book. And, despite many of these practices involving quiet, meditative time for visioning, you do not have to be a hermit in a cave, meditating hour after hour. You can be a regular human expanding your life and vitality and control over your physical, mental, and spiritual body, helping you to feel less helpless and more capable and confident, and to begin again to look forward to starting each day.

True, with a health challenge, not everyone can start their healing journey as easily as Jill did; however, with the help of the techniques and practices I teach in this book, you can learn to move from fear to living with an upbeat attitude, in charge of your personal journey no matter what your health and wellness challenges.

Studying shamanism taught me elements that also will be key for you in your learning. To gain greater knowledge about how to move forward with any life challenge, you will need to have greater intuition about the possibilities available to you. I never considered myself intuitive until I started working with energy and doing the practices I teach here. Since then, my intuition has grown, or at the very least, I have improved my ability to listen to the more subtle messages.

It's also critical to learn about the power of the mind. We have been shown that our thoughts influence our energy fields and thus how our lives play out. In this way, when we make our thoughts clearer, when we more accurately express our desires, that increased refinement of our thoughts impacts the outcome of our fields, and hence our lives. My intuition serves me well in my medical practice even though my medical training did not encourage me to pay attention to messages from my gut.

I remember the time when a frail, elderly man came in for his appointment, still shaken from the very recent death of his wife. I stopped just before beginning my usual rundown on blood pressure and cholesterol lab readings. Something "told" me to ask him if his wife was still "around." At first, he looked surprised, but despite my unusual query, he did not waste a moment telling me that a few days before, he walked by their closet and smelled violets, her favorite flower. What is more, every evening, his little dog would go into the sunroom and jump up and down as if waiting for his wife to grab his leash and get ready to walk him as she had regularly done when she was still alive. So here the dog was, weeks after her death, jumping up and down alongside something invisible. Another day, soon after her death, my patient had come back from the store and found their wedding photo on the sideboard, which caught him completely off guard as the photo had been put away in a box for years.

"It was so strange. I couldn't explain how it could possibly have gotten there!" he said. But he then reflected that he felt comforted realizing she had moved the photo to send him a sign.

Listening when something "told" me to switch gears from "running the numbers" (focusing on the values of blood pressure readings or blood sugars) to talking about the unseen world opened the door to a powerful conversation that was healing for this grieving patient. I shared with him that I believe that a person's soul can exist after life and that we can receive messages from the afterlife in ways we cannot explain. I told him that although science cannot explain these occurrences, I find them to be real. He told me it was good to talk about these topics. He seemed comforted by our discussion.

It took a lot of courage for me to talk to patients about the new ways of seeing that shamanism has shown me. I was afraid of discussing any ideas that were not based in data-defined, scientifically backed concepts; therefore, bringing up the idea that a dead person could still have a presence and talking aloud to a patient about this was a bold step for me.

For a while, I was temporarily locked in a box that constrained my office life to the standards of care of Western medicine, but after several similar spiritual discussions and seeing how easily patients resonate with talking about energy and spirit, I felt liberated. I no longer hold back out of fear of not being considered a "real" doctor.

From that time on, I began to speak more openly about my new way of seeing illness and how it impacts the life journey. I now speak to patients either directly or with metaphors about where they find themselves on their soul's journey (in this lifetime) and whether this is how they wish to live. When patients are approached this way, particularly during chronic debilitation, a spark is lit. Patients see themselves from the higher vantage point—one of a soul essence on a human journey—and can tap into their reserves of courage and commitment to find a new approach to their health challenge.

Integrating traditional Western medicine and shamanism gives me broader tools with which to guide change for my patients. Let us take diabetes as an example. Diabetes is a disease that requires a lot of involvement on the part of the patient. My Western medical approach will continue to focus on blood sugars to improve diabetic control, but now I can add my shamanic approach.

I might start talking about how a patient sees his future life and what he sees as the reason for his resistance to taking control (that is, not testing his sugars as advised). I would share my intuitions of where I "see" the stagnation of life force in his energy field. I might then suggest what the patient could do spiritually or with ritual to help shift his resistance and to clear that stagnation. Not all patients are open to this; some think it is nonsense, just as they think coming to the doctor several times a year is nonsense. However, if just one patient is moved to change for the better, then I am happy.

As you walk with me, you will learn to broaden your view of yourself, of the world, and of your place in the world. You will start to "see" your energy field and learn how to make it more vital. You will connect with the Universal Field and its forces and become more adept at communicating with the unseen world. I will teach you how to enhance your intuition, have integrity of thought, and visualize your future. These teachings will bring you to a place of greater clarity, wisdom, and power for the purpose of your transformation and the transformation of any health challenge that may arise.

Why Western Medicine
Is Not Enough

The scientific world of Western medicine, in which I had my core training as a physician, is a healing system that includes the understanding of parts of the human organism ranging from entire organ systems to individual cells and their parts. Western medicine uses "rational therapeutics" to treat disease, looking at biochemical processes that have gone awry and using medications designed to interact within those processes with the goal of restoring normal functioning.

For example, chemotherapy to treat cancer employs some astonishingly clever medications. Monoclonal antibodies attack cancer cells' defense system. Other medications prevent blood vessel growth, causing cancer cells to be starved of nutrients and subsequently die. Western medicine is increasingly precise in affecting cellular processes and is moving toward targeted therapeutics, whereby medications are chosen based on the patient's unique genetic makeup. As a former research scientist, I applaud these discoveries. Some of the advances in treatment are nothing short of miraculous.

By all accounts, Western medicine is brilliant, and I want to acknowledge its benefits. Unlike in the past, we are no longer losing our children as infants, and we now have available to us remarkable surgeries such as hip replacement, kidney transplant, and open heart surgery. In America, the life expectancy was around 39 years in 1860 and was almost double that in 2020. These advances are amazing.

Western medicine was not always high tech nor sophisticated, however. It took a lot of time for physicians to learn from observation and trials what worked to improve health or prevent disease.

Imagine that the year is 1795. Smallpox is rampant across what is now called the United Kingdom. People didn't realize the disease is caused by a virus that is spread easily by droplets from someone coughing or from blister fluid; babies were easily infected. Infected people developed a fever, rash, blisters, nausea, and vomiting, and some of those that lived developed severe scarring where the blisters were, even blindness. If they were unlucky (around 3 in 10 people), they experienced organ collapse and death. In fact, about 400,000 people a year died of smallpox.

In England, a country doctor named Edward Jenner was treating smallpox patients. He observed that many of the milkmaids who got blisters from working with cows (cowpox) did not catch smallpox. Dr. Jenner decided to try something new—he scratched the arm of a young boy and placed blister fluid from cowpox into the scratch, in effect exposing the boy to cowpox virus. The boy got a localized blister (the result of being infected with a mild form of cowpox). After being infected with this milder virus, Dr. Jenner then scratched the boy's arm with blister fluid from a smallpox blister, and the boy did not catch smallpox! The technique spread, and soon many people were having their arms scratched, an early form of vaccination. Jenner is credited with being the father of vaccination. Now, in all accuracy, when I researched vaccination history, China and the Middle East were using similar forms of vaccination hundreds of years prior to Jenner. Regardless, thanks to vaccination, in 1980, naturally occurring smallpox was considered eradicated.

Before the mid-1900s, Western medicine had limits that might seem unimaginable today. Anesthesia was crude or nonexistent in the 1800s, and surgeries themselves were barbaric. During the Civil War, 600,000 amputations were performed, mostly from limbs damaged by rifles. Because of the risk of life-threatening infections, limbs were amputated to save the soldiers' lives. The best doctor was one who could saw off your leg fastest, often in the absence of anesthesia.

At the same time as battlefield operations were going on in rough fashion, medical advances were being made in the use of anesthesia. Rudimentary forms of anesthesia, such as drinking boiled herbs with cannabis or opium, had been used for centuries, but in 1846, a demonstration of ether as an anesthetic was carried out at Massachusetts General Hospital in Boston. Despite the poor efficacy of ether (the patients told of ongoing pain when they woke up), its use did markedly change the experience of a surgical operation.

Medical advances kept coming, as physicians and scientists applied knowledge of biology, physiology, and physics to medicine. The physicist Roentgen invented X-rays in the late 1800s, and by the 1950s, they were being used for medical diagnosis. Louis Pasteur showed the scientific world how germs were spread, and in 1847, a Hungarian surgeon named Semmelweis instituted handwashing procedures on his surgical wards, dramatically cutting down on post-operative infections. In 1928, Alexander Fleming found that a mold stopped bacteria from growing in a lab petri dish, and during World War II, this mold, known as penicillin, was mass produced, saving many people from death due to bacterial infections. Anesthesia was improved, and we have many forms, from a rapid on-and-off infusion of propofol, to localized nerve blocks, to various forms of inhaled gases. Specialized training in anesthesia is taught in universities; it is almost unheard of for a patient to say they felt any pain during an operation.

Western medicine has accomplished significant advances in discovering insulin, fighting infection, and using targeted pharmaceuticals for what are mostly Western conditions: high blood pressure, chronic pulmonary disease, heart disease, and diabetes. Surgery has become more sophisticated, too. Surgeons can perform complex gamma knife brain surgery and even organ transplants.

The extraordinary accomplishments of Western medicine can also be seen in the use of medical devices that are used externally or implanted. Even after months on respiratory support (ventilator), patients with COVID pneumonia can often be discharged from the hospital. Many people are living longer because of Western medicine.

On the other hand, Western medicine is fraught with limitations, which I recognized way back when I was first in medical school.

Comparing Western Medicine and Maximum Medicine

Over the years, I have watched as people have become increasingly frustrated with Western medicine and flocked to the offerings of alternative and integrative medicine. I wonder if the draw to alternative healing is not the result of something simple: Western medicine points out what is "wrong" (in lab results, in X-ray findings) while alternative medicine advertises how a person can be "more" or experience what is "super" (superfoods, superimmunity).

In other words, Western medicine sees people as becoming increasingly defective as years go by and offers ways to try to restore people toward (but never reaching) their baseline. Alternative or complementary medicine promises functionality above the average, beyond deficits. A 2016 *New York Times* article reported that Americans spend $30 billion on alternative or complementary health care. Something is pulling people away from Western medicine. I suspect the flaws I see in it have been observed by everyday people, too, as they interact with our health care system.

When I first took a class in shamanic healing—and truthfully, in every other alternative healing workshop or teaching I have attended—I heard conversations about how much the attendees (and by extension, all people) hate doctors. Picture it: I am sitting next to my classmates as they talk about how clueless physicians are, how doctors never consider the energetics of a situation, how doctors never listen, and the list goes on. I don't argue out loud, but in my mind, I say, *That's not true. I get it. And I know I am not the only physician that does.*

In today's Western medicine, particularly in hospitals, patients' opinions are gathered to determine whether the doctor communicated well, whether the nurse listened about the patients' pain, whether medication side effects were explained. The result on these surveys is tied to government reimbursement. Believe me when I tell you that in every hospital I have worked, scores are never high. I personally believe that the dissatisfaction starts before a patient even gets admitted to a hospital and exists independently of these surveys.

So if many are dissatisfied, why is the change so terribly slow? I and others are envisioning a change, however long it takes to bring about: We want Maximum Medicine for all. What if taking care of patients could incorporate not only the latest treatments but the best of all that came before?

Bringing Back Indigenous and Shamanistic Ways of Healing

As Western medicine became more popular, traditional treatments that had been handed down for generations were cast aside, despite the benefits of some of those approaches. We relegated much of what was valuable in ancient medicine to the realm of snake oil, meaning it was considered fraudulent and hyped only by charlatans. In doing that, we lost a lot.

For one thing, healing practitioners no longer employed the healing power of plants and using food as medicine. The value of a plant-based diet in healing the typical Western diseases of inflammation and atherosclerosis is indisputable. Pharmaceuticals are brilliant in their ability to target a specific enzyme pathway or chemical in the body; however, they often have side effects, some of which can be not just inconvenient but dangerous. Sometimes, the chemical reaction is so narrowly targeted that while the medication helps one part of the body, it harms another. Having evolved alongside us over millennia, plants might provide a broader chemical synergy with our bodies and thus, a smoother healing process.

By its very nature, Western medicine necessitates the use of prescription drugs. These can be extremely expensive and, as I said, they often come with side effects. At the same time that patients are increasingly being given more choices for prescription medications, they are becoming less autonomous and taking less responsibility for their health, particularly in the areas of nutrition and exercise. It seems that the physicians who advocate for nutrition as medicine, who promote ways to prevent disease by what you eat and by adopting healthy lifestyle habits, are in the minority. (Drs. Joel Fuhrman, Dean Ornish, Mark Hyman, and others come to mind, as well as other functional or integrative medicine physicians.)

Shamans traditionally used plant medicine in another way, too: They ingested certain medicinal plants to go into shamanic trances and take psychogenic journeys, allowing them to access a deeper state of knowledge about the cause of the illness and the type of treatment and healing an individual needed. In shamanism, it's believed that disease can be caused by harmful energies or actions that person has taken. Getting to the source of that energetic influence can lead to healing. Too often, Western medicine dismisses insights that can be gained through going beyond the limitations of the conscious, analytical mind to access wisdom greater than our own.

Today's physicians typically don't look to the root source of illness, and they often completely disregard intuition. Hunches about the cause of suffering aren't considered evidence-based medicine. Physicians will typically not set an intention to harness every healing tool available—pharmaceutical drugs and surgery but also spirituality, the patients' consciousness, and the universal energy field. They don't apply the spiritual approaches of prayer and divination to seek divine guidance for the patient. Gone is the foremost understanding in indigenous ways—that Spirit, Nature, and the unseen world play integral roles in healing.

Shamanism is an approach to healing that, unlike Western medicine or energy medicine (an approach I'll explain more about later), is also a way of being, intricately linking the practitioner to the essences and forces of all things, animate and inanimate, including forces of Nature. To the shaman or shamanic practitioner, all things in Nature—trees, animals, weather, stones, water, sky, and so on—are intimately connected, each interacting and dependent on each other and imbued with a spiritual energy or force. These forces impact the geographic locale, as well as the community and the individual, and thus must be considered and reckoned with. The shamanic practitioner is skilled at divining for the one seeking healing and changing the course of that client's life path by negotiating with "spirits" (unseen forces).

In most cultures that include shamanism as part of their traditions, the healers go into altered states of consciousness (by chanting, dancing, drumming, or with use of psychogenic plants) to access knowledge from the unseen world, including insights offered from "spirits." The knowledge is used not just for healing an individual but to guide decisions of the community: whether to move their camp to another location, where to fish or hunt, or how to help a person heal, including which plants to use and which spirits (forces) to fight against. Shamanic interaction with unseen forces is also used to change the weather and the community's fortune.

When their intention is to help an individual heal, shamans enter a trance, as I said, or they use prayer or dreamtime (accessing universal knowledge through dream visions) so their consciousness can interact with the quantum or universal energy field. Shamanic healers believe that there is no separation throughout the universe—that every being and everything that exists, did exist, or will exist is a part of this vast energy matrix, a vibratory field in which every thought and every action has consequences.

In Lynne McTaggart's *The Field: The Quest for the Secret Force of the Universe,* she writes:

> If a quantum field holds us all together in its invisible web, we will have to rethink our definitions of ourselves and what exactly it is to be human. If we are in constant and instantaneous dialogue with our environment, if all the information from the cosmos flows through our pores at every moment, then our current notion of our human potential is only a glimmer of what it should be.[4]

Shamans work holistically by not just treating the physical body as Western doctors do but also the emotions, thoughts, and the spirit of the individual they are helping. Shamans do all of this by accessing the universal matrix. In Western medicine, it's unusual for physicians to set an intention to harness every healing tool available—not just pharmaceutical drugs and surgery but also the universal energy field as well as their own spirituality and their patient's consciousness.

In contrast, shamans work to create shifts in the trajectory of the client's health by interacting with what they find in the Universal Field, which can even include ancestral knowledge. Ancestors, even when deceased, are believed to be guiding individuals and can be turned to (in dreams or ritual practice) for answers and wisdom.

Some providers in Western medicine (such as psychologists and psychiatrists) might argue that they work with the wisdom and knowledge of the ancestors, in the sense that a mental health professional might have you imagine a conversation with your grandmother to learn more about the origin of a trait or habit of yours. However, a shaman can access forgotten family history, along with knowledge offered by ancestors other than your own.

Indigenous healers recognize that healing comes not just from medications or surgeries but from connection to energies of Nature (wind, thunder, lightning, flood), in concert with the seasons, the sun, moon, and stars, and the life cycles of plants and animals. The forces of Nature are revered as sacred. Among most indigenous cultures, the healers are also the priests or spiritual leaders and often herbalists who are well versed in the use of plant medicine. In the West, our healers are rarely spiritual leaders.

What's more, in indigenous healing, which works with the Universal Field we all share, the patient is not seen as separate from the community but as an integral part. In many cultures, the perspective is that if one person is ill, the entire community is affected. The vitality of one is considered as essential to the health of all. As Western medicine became more popular, the holistic view of each patient within her group, with her unique purpose to her community, was discarded.

I personally am committed to the whole of the patient; I believe engaging that whole can yield more powerful healing. At first, my belief simmered below the surface of my day-to-day actions; I had no "proof" of the power of engaging the whole. After studying shamanism and experiencing the shifts that could occur when all realms (literal, emotional, spiritual, energetic) were worked with, I was more strongly committed to the holistic view.

Western medicine has moved away from viewing patients holistically; in other words, considering how the mind, body, and spirit interact in health and disease. Instead, physicians are locked into short office visits, with costs billed to insurance companies. This practice favors a volume of patients over the quality of the interaction with each individual and links medicine to finances.

That puts physicians in a difficult position, creating a huge conflict of interest when treatment options are being considered. Often left behind in modern Western medical practice is spending time talking to the patient, understanding the family dynamics that affect the individual's health, and recognizing the role of the patient's spirituality. Doctors too often have little time to teach patients how to make changes that can alter the course of their health. Not many people hold the beliefs I do: that they have considerable capacity to heal themselves and can learn how to do it.

Also, shamanism is ritualistic. Examples include using a fire to communicate with spirits, drumming or using a rattle to evoke an altered state, or preparing a herbal brew in a particular way. Western practitioners may have personal rituals, such as praying before beginning an operation or starting their workday, but this isn't the norm. That's unfortunate, because when you perform a ritual, you are blocking distractions, going inward, and connecting to your God, your inner self, and the energy field that integrates you. If the ritual is one performed by many people over time, you are contributing to building a vortex of power.

I believe we tap into a collective memory about rituals. If we're in a sacred site, a place where rituals were held for millennia, standing where others stood, we connect with and activate an energetic memory of the rituals performed there by people who share our state of mind and our intention. This sacred shift allows us to feel our interconnection with the sacred and with the Universal Field, where we can attain the knowledge we seek.

About the Evidence

Unfortunately, we do not have a lot of recordings of healing practices used among indigenous populations that document effective healing treatments, which would be helpful for data-gathering purposes. Most healing expertise was handed down from generation to generation, from village herbalist and day keeper or mountain medicine man to their apprentices.

The healer-in-training assisted the expert and carefully observed the diagnosis and treatment processes. Because the knowledge has been transmitted orally and experientially, it can be difficult to understand exactly how a shaman "sees" the illness or how she accesses the "cure."

I believe that as more shamanic traditions are brought forth to the modern world by practitioners who can bridge language and cultural gaps, we will see that shamanic medicine incorporates what many would call "energy medicine" (more on that topic shortly). Whether each culture's shamans would say they see chakras (energy funnels/centers that are attached to the body) or the luminous energy field will remain to be seen.

What we do have are glimpses of various unique forms of healing that incorporated mind, body, and spirit. These included divination techniques to access hidden wisdom—for example, in African traditions, healers would shake and throw bones for divination, intuiting the meaning of the arrangement. Other forms of healing involved brushing the client with herbs (limpia, as practiced in Central America) and having people cleanse themselves with burning sage ("smudging," as practiced in North America) or by using a sweat lodge ceremony.

Many traditions used prayers and rituals for healing that, in a lot of cases, became lost to history.

One great indigenous healer whose methods were documented was Frank Fools Crow. Fools Crow was a Lakota elder, resident of the Pine Ridge Reservation in South Dakota. By any standards, indigenous or modern, his healings were miraculous and legendary. Thomas E. Mails, author of *Fools Crow: Wisdom and Power,* documented times when Fools Crow would be in prayer and manifest (bring forth in form) stones that traveled into a patient's lungs. When Frank pulled the stones out, the infection would come as well.[5]

Fools Crow worked within the spiritual realm, with prayer and close connection to unseen forces of Nature, to elicit the healings that he did. Even so, we don't understand the mechanisms by which these healings occurred, so we have to rely on the testament of patients and witnesses to the shamanic medicine he used.

In traditional shamanism, when the shaman does a journey (an experience undertaken while in an altered state awareness to access unseen wisdom and forces), he is using his power of thought and awareness to access universal knowledge and intelligence and bringing those to bear on a client's future. The client, meanwhile, might be holding a positivity of thought to visualize a healed outcome. This power of directed thought is key to successful outcomes.

Frank Fools Crow was asked by Thomas Mails why he had his client come and spend four days in his teepee. Did it take four days for Frank's medicine to work? Fools Crow explained to his biographer that the power of his medicine was instantaneous but that four days were needed for the client to get right for the medicine to work.[6]

In my interpretation of this, he meant that the client must believe in a successful outcome and be prepared and open to receive the healing. Both healing approaches show success by how the client "feels," and generally that improved "feeling" is shown by improvement in behaviors or symptoms.

In my personal experience, shamanic and energy techniques are extremely powerful as judged by how the clients feel after a session. Nearly 100 percent of my shamanic clients feel better nearly immediately, and the feeling is long lasting. I have never experienced a traditional Western medicine approach to be this efficacious or well received. In shamanic medicine, results are not easily observed, measured, or quantified. Shamanic practitioners will tell you that in their clients, pain disappears, illnesses drop away, and clients act on new choices in their lives, leading to lasting changes in not only illness but the experience of being sick. So, in this sense, more weight is put on a sense of being "healed" as opposed to being "cured." The client feels better and can navigate life better regardless of the actual physical healing (for example, whether the cancer has been removed).

Can Western Medicine Change?

What we are just starting to recognize in Western medicine is that people don't have bodies that behave like machines that need to be maintained and then, when they fall into a state of disrepair, fixed. People's emotions and thoughts (consciousness) strongly impact their health and ability to heal, and the patient's intention regarding healing powerfully affects the outcome of any health interventions.

I would also argue that the belief of the practitioner plays a key role in Western medicine, even though it is rarely acknowledged, studied, or commented on. If a physician decides that the findings on a lung scan indicate spots of cancer, the subsequent discussion with the patient and the unfolding path of testing and referral to specialists becomes fixed under the belief that only a bad outcome is possible. But if a physician holds in her mind the possibility that the spots are a treatable inflammatory condition, the path prescribed is much different.

Western medicine addresses this dilemma by encouraging a provider to create a "differential diagnosis," holding in their mind multiple possibilities, not just one. This list of possibilities only creates a diverse testing plan; it does not often translate into the provider carrying a belief of a good outcome for the patient.

Fortunately, many modern-day physicians have begun to recognize the power of the words they use and the words the patient chooses to use to describe a medical challenge. Consider the differences between "Mrs. Jones, your lung scan shows a mass, which is probably cancerous. The next step is to set you up for a biopsy. What day works best for you?" versus "Mrs. Jones, unfortunately your lung scan shows a mass. It could be any number of things, from cancer to a benign tumor to a fungal infection to an overgrowth of blood vessels. We will plan to do a biopsy, and depending on the results, we will make a treatment plan. Whatever the mass turns out to be, we will work through this together."

The first statement is accurate and guides a testing course, but it offers nothing that sounds remotely like hope. The second statement leaves open the possibility for something other than cancer and reminds the patient that they are not alone in facing the results of the testing and any treatment decisions to be made. In which scenario do you think the patient leaves the office with some light shining in the tunnel? Which scenario amplifies positivity and brings in hope?

Energy Medicine

Given the limitations of Western medicine, let's consider not just shamanic medicine, which in its purest form has been around for 30,000 years; let's also look at "energy medicine," a term coined in the 1980s to describe any informational or energetic interaction to restore balance and harmony to the client. Understanding energy medicine can better help you understand how shamanic practitioners work with energy fields to bring about healing.

In 1988, Richard Gerber, M.D., published a ground-breaking book, *Vibrational Medicine,* in which he described vibrational medicine and techniques using the subtle energies of the body.[7] He was one of the first people—and certainly one of the first physicians—to talk about energy medicine and working directly with energy fields.

In general, his healing approach focuses on restoring balance to different parts of the body by working with energy fields to adjust their frequencies, using crystals, tuning forks, and the hands. He wrote about using magnets, colors (which have different wavelengths of light), and frequencies of sounds for the purpose of bringing back the body and its organs and systems into a natural state of balance.

He also wrote about the flow of chi, or life force, along acupuncture meridians and within chakras. Working with these subtle psychic energy centers of the body—energy funnels or vortexes that extend outward from the body and are part of the luminous energy field—is at the core of the practice of energy medicine.

Some energy medicine practitioners, such as Anodea Judith, who wrote *Charge and the Energy Body,* track the energy of the chakra centers.[8] First written about in Hindu scriptures around 500 BC, chakras have typically been interpreted by modern energy medicine practitioners as being linked to endocrine and organ systems; however, this direct link was not identified in ancient writings.

In addition to practitioners who use chakra work, there are some, such as Gerber and chiropractor Carolyn McMakin, who take a vibrational energy approach. In her book *The Resonance Effect: How Frequency Specific Microcurrent Is Changing Medicine,* Dr. McMakin describes her process of placing electrodes on her client and applying an electrical current of a certain frequency and getting reduction of pain, release of tight muscle groups and even decreased time to healing. She also tells a story of treating a professional football player who had broken his leg. As expected, after surgery, the leg was swollen and bruised and painful. She applied particular frequencies (using electrodes and a machine to generate current). The swelling decreased, bruising resolved, and pain went away in a very short time—much shorter than was expected from traditional recovery times.[9]

There are many forms of energy medicine, including reiki and Healing Touch. Inherent in all these approaches is the belief that there is a universal, intelligent energy field to which all individual beings are connected, a belief found in Hindu and Buddhist mysticism. Many say that our thoughts connect us to the Universal Field and its transpersonal realms, which we can't necessarily see or sense when we're in an ordinary state of consciousness but that anyone potentially can travel to with their consciousness. Energy medicine practitioners say that subtle energies of the body can be shifted through the power of thought (usually their own cohesive, focused thoughts). As all things are interconnected, a practitioner can connect her consciousness to that Universal Field and thus connect to the field of the client. In this way, the practitioner can shift the energetic frequencies of the client and entrain them to a changed, healed state.

The key approach to healing using energy medicine involves positive thoughts or intentions (focused aim). Thoughts have power. When I see a spot on a lung X-ray, I call on the field around me, which connects my patient and me, to entrain itself to my belief that what I'm looking at is as harmless as can be. Of course, if a lung biopsy were to prove it is something malignant, I'll discuss treatments, but initially, I choose to maintain the most powerfully positive thought that I can. Whenever you create a thought, you affect the energy field we all share. I want to be sure I'm affecting it in the best possible way.

According to energy medicine practitioners, all life experiences change an individual's energy field. Harsh words directed at you, or actual physical trauma, leave lasting changes (imprints) in the field; the field is then damaged, becoming congested and less free flowing, which gives rise to a potential for illness in the same way that a physical trauma, such as a surgery or injury, can. An energy medicine practitioner uses their consciousness and intention to remove any blocks and restore flow in the energy field and action. Also, while acupuncture, which uses needles, may be stimulating the nervous system, which in turn brings about changes in the body, some would say it also affects the flow of chi, or life force, to bring about balance and healing, giving it similarities to energy medicine.

While I have read much about energy medicine and incorporate it into my work, it's my shamanic training that gives me context for the value of interacting with energy fields that affect the human body.

My Shamanic Training

The "shamanism" I have trained in is not that of the throat singers of Mongolia, the shamans who take canoe journeys to the Underworld, or the ones who drink a mind-altering brew from the ayahuascaros, although I fully accept that these traditions have immense power. What I mean is that I did not apprentice in these styles, and thus do not routinely connect to wind horses, or to underworld beings, or go into psychedelic trances. I learned a shamanism with origins in the Andes, arguably a modernized shamanism related to that of the masked, drumming practitioners of Siberia.

My shamanism recognizes the unseen world of Spirit, that Spirit can be connected and conversed with, and that human consciousness can explore the vibratory world of the universal energy matrix and encourage those energies to change based on personal intention. For me, the world of Spirit (which is in and of itself an energy world) has immense power; this resource can be harnessed to bring more control over our lives and our destiny. So, for me, shamanism is using techniques to access Spirit and the matrix of the Universal Field and applying that to the healing of myself and others.

I do not follow a straight lineage, such as that of the Andean light workers or !Kung bushmen. Rather, I will mix anything that allows me and others to gain awareness of our energy field and consciousness and even link up with the very real forces of the earth, galaxy, and universe. These forces can be encouraged to be allies, and when we cultivate a relationship, we have access to an immense reservoir of empowerment.

I have studied energy medicine, and I include what I've learned in how I work with patients. What I call Maximum Medicine includes many ways of the indigenous, including the mystical and spiritual, while recognizing and using glorious, scientific knowledge. When viewed as a three-circle Venn diagram, the center where Western medicine, energy medicine, and shamanic rituals blend and overlap is, to me, a focal point of immense understanding of human beings and great potency for healing.

One of the reasons I deeply respect indigenous, shamanic medicine for is that in these traditions, healing is sustainable, meaning that there is no limit to the availability of the methods and tools used to restore or improve health and wellness. Unless a person is incapable of thought, they can work with dreamtime, prayer, and rituals. With or without a shaman's help, a person can tap into universal consciousness and the universal matrix.

Another reason I embrace shamanic medicine is because it has no shelf life and no patents or trademarks. This contrasts with Western medical treatments using pharmaceuticals. Depending on how recently the medicine was invented it might be very costly, and thus inaccessible to many patients. Surgery and even preventive care can be costly, too.

Western medicine practitioners will often work with their patients to make healthcare more affordable and accessible, and I applaud my colleagues who make these efforts, but we have a long way to go to match the availability and affordability of treatment offered by shamanic medicine. I feel that in order to maximize medicine, it's important to use energy medicine and shamanic medicine and to bring back the mystical.

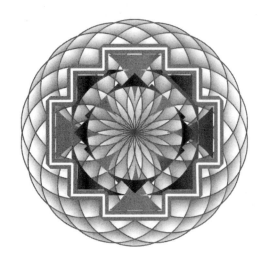

Part Two
———————

MAXIMUM
MEDICINE
FUNDAMENTALS

Bring Back the Mystical

Over the years, I have explored the mystical mainly for myself and not related to my role as a physician healer. I was open to spirits surviving after death, to the existence of another dimension in which spirits of those who had passed on lived. My sister experienced waking up in the middle of the night and seeing our great uncle standing at her bedside. Later, in the morning, she received a phone call from his wife, our great aunt, saying my great uncle had passed away at the same time my sister had seen him.

Hearing her story about how Uncle Walker came to her in the middle of the night did not shock or distress me; I was completely receptive to it. I had read stories of Edgar Cayce's experiences, explored reincarnation through my reading, and had lived in Thailand, where I learned about Buddhism, so this way of sensing other dimensions beyond our tangible world was acceptable to me.

In my shamanic training, during our visualizations (journeys), my classmates and I had experiences of seeing and knowing things about the others that we had no way of knowing, at least, from the literal world perspective. Often, these phenomena occurred while we were performing shamanic rituals. In that environment, we accepted the validity of the unseen world. Let me share an example.

Early in our shamanic training, I and my classmates were working with the three stones we each had been asked to bring to the workshop. We were learning how to develop our intuition using our stones. For one exercise, we gathered into groups of two and were instructed to work closely with a partner. Our task was to hold one of our stones and then "read" the stone, meaning discern, intuit, or "know" some information about our partner while holding our stone.

I picked up one of my stones, a gray-and-brown stone with one small white line running through it. The stone was completely nondescript, if I am being truthful. I remember willing myself to drop out of my logical mind into a place of receiving information from my inner self. I did not have experience doing this, but I told my analytic brain to be quiet and searched my awareness for another source of knowledge.

Next, I rubbed my stone over my third eye (the spot between the eyebrows), knowing that this energy center, also called the mind's eye or inner eye, is recognized as a mystical, invisible eye that provides perception beyond ordinary sight. The third eye is said to be the gate that leads to the inner realms and spaces of higher consciousness. I then brought the stone into my left hand and began focusing my attention by rubbing the stone between my thumb and first finger.

I should tell you that I had never met my practice partner before this workshop, and had yet to work with her in the workshop, so I was going in blind. Well, maybe not! As I looked at the stone, I saw a drawing of a large boat moving across the flat surface of the stone to the left. The waves were high and tumultuous. I sensed fear and panic. And I saw that on the left side of the "screen" of the stone face, the sun was shining and the world was calmer.

I quieted my logical mind, which was screaming at me, *You are making this up! You can't see anything. If you tell her this, she will think you are a wacko,* and told my partner what I had "seen."

"You are in a boat in stormy seas, and you are scared. You are afraid you are going to sink, but do not worry—your ship is leaving the storm, and the seas are quiet ahead. You will be okay."

Sitting nervously, waiting for her to look at me as if I were crazy, I realized she was crying. She told me that she was in a very bad time in her life. She was getting a divorce, moving, and in need of a new job. She also told me that she had had a dream a few nights prior that she was on a boat rocked by huge waves and that, in the dream, she had feared she would capsize. Imagine both of our amazement at the depth of this interconnected experience! Imagine our excitement at tasting how to tap into our intuitive, shamanic, and energetic capacities!

Hours later, the clear image of the boat and seas was not visible on the face of the stone, although I had the awareness of that vision. A few months later, as I lifted that stone, I could no longer see anything resembling the story, and could not even conjure up a similar interpretation; there are no lines or marks on the stone to offer such!

A few years after starting my shamanic training, I gathered up the courage to start talking to my patients about things outside the scope of Western medicine. My mind was filled with worries about whether the discussions were outside of "standard of care" and whether I could talk using my spiritual paradigms in a neighborhood filled with fundamentalist Christians. Little by little, I began introducing the idea of unseen influences on health.

One time, I had a young woman come to me complaining of fatigue and exhaustion that was expressed mostly in her body as back pain. First, following my default approach, using the first of the three circles in the Venn diagram, I did a Western medicine workup. When this workup was found to be unrevealing in Western medicine terms, I stepped into the other two circles of awareness—those of energy and shamanism.

When I sensed her back pain and her overall vitality, I could sense her being burdened, often by her own doing, taking on more than her share of responsibility. I offered to her that I saw her back pain as an extra burden and wondered why she might be carrying so much.

I then wondered to myself if she were operating under what shamans call a "soul contract," one in which she had agreed to "carry the load." A soul contract is felt to be an agreement that the soul makes prior to incarnation, in relation to other souls, as to how to behave in the literal world. Or, as Danielle MacKinnon wrote in her book *Soul Contracts:*

> Born out of despair, fear, pain, or anger, a soul contract is an unconscious promise that you've made with yourself in the past that is now hindering your ability to move forward in life.[10]

I asked this young woman, "Do you always have to be the one who does everything?"

Tearfully, she said, "Yes. It's my job."

I responded, "Does it feel like too much to carry?"

"Yes, I am tired of doing it all."

I then said, "Who said you have to do this?"

She answered, "It's always been that way."

I then proceeded to tell her that what I was about to share had no known explanation in scientific medicine, but rather came from my spiritual beliefs. I told her that I believed souls came to this earth with contracts ("rules") from past lifetimes that influence our health and well-being.[11] She was listening intently, absorbing everything I said.

I continued, "Your contract to take it all on as your duty is adding to your back pain. I can show you a way to get out from under that rule."

She nodded, crying. I then taught her a visualization to use, one in which she would go before God or her Higher Self or spirit guides and express her desire for a new contract. When I saw her back in the office a few weeks later, she had done the practice. She reported that her pain was markedly improved, she was feeling lighter and more upbeat.

I was happy because, in this case, there was no good fix in the Western medicine part of the Venn diagram for lower back pain when X-rays show there are no pinched nerves or deteriorated discs. Western medicine can offer pain pills, physical therapy, spinal injections, or "just live with it." Now, however, I have something else to offer: spiritual and energetic approaches that I believe have longer-lasting benefits, with less cost and fewer side effects.

What I learned from this encounter is that when I, a Western-trained physician, began to speak from alternative perspectives (spiritual, energetic, and shamanistic), my patients responded positively. This young woman was not the only patient with whom I talked "differently." I was able to become more and more confident in being able to offer patients a new approach to healing, and more and more, I sought to work from the center of the Maximum Medicine Venn diagram.

Learning Basic Shamanic and Energy Medicine Practices

In the chapters that follow, I will teach you the basic elements of the energy field and some shamanic techniques and show you how to apply these to a personal or health challenge. Irrespective of seeking to fix something, these techniques and practices are an amazing, robust way to expand your consciousness and amplify your personal power in the world. Your experience of life will grow fuller, you will gain vitality, and you will get more clarity on making life decisions as they arise.

To achieve these goals, you need to begin experiencing your connection with the invisible world and the messages it has for you. Throughout this book, you will find several meditations like the one that follows. Each has components that are integral to the journeys you will take.

You may record the visualizations in this book in your voice, then use the recordings to play back to yourself. This might help you to deepen, leaving your planning thoughts and analytical brain behind.

◊ In every visualization exercise, you will start from an internal place of sacredness as well as a particular geographic place that might in time become "your" place. As you will learn in chapter 12, these locations or sacred spaces can be inside your house or outside in nature. The more you sit in sacred moments (in prayer or quiet time or meditation) in these spaces, the more you will build their power and the more special these spaces will become for you.

◊ No matter what physical space I'm in when I do visualizations, I like to start all journeys, unless a different way is specified, by drawing my awareness to my heart space. Visualizing from the heart helps move me out of my active, literal mind and allows my awareness to be freer and more fluid.

◊ You will have a journal and pen and/or drawing materials nearby to record important awarenesses that arise during the journey.

◊ You will declare the work you will do as sacred. This means you put "all" of you into the process: your thoughts, your deepest desires, your commitment, your promise to yourself to work at the changes the process shows you. You will set an intention to enter an inner sacred space to connect with Spirit—and perhaps also with spiritual allies (a topic we'll explore later in this book).

◊ You may ask for spiritual allies (spirit guides, angels, power animals) to join you in the work. If your spirit helpers choose not to come with you on a specific occasion, not to worry— Spirit and your helpers know what is best for you at any given time. (Later, you'll learn about invoking Spirit and helpers when seeking their assistance. I do this as part of opening sacred space, setting my intention to work within it.)

◊ During your interactions with Spirit and any holy beings, you will ask for their input and their agreement. This is a key component of being in *ayni* (EYE-nee), a Quechuan term for "right relationship." (Quechua is the language spoken by the Andean shamans of the Q'ero people who trained me in shamanic wisdom and techniques.) A balance of give and take makes for respectful alliances.

◊ You will sit quietly and take a few deep breaths, allowing your muscles and belly to relax. Relax long enough to leave behind the strong influence and heavy activity of your conscious mind and enter your subconscious space. Much like with hypnosis, you will entertain ideas or statements that reach and affect your subconscious, making more of an impact on what you think or believe deep down and what you experience.

◊ You will take your awareness on a visualization, or journey; that is, you will use your mind's eye to see an image, and you'll step into that image with your essence, your awareness. If you have difficulty visualizing, allow your inner ear or inner knowing to communicate with you.

◊ You will take yourself where you wish to go to gain knowledge or to instruct a change, exploring the territory that opens up to you when you have calmed your conscious mind with its rational thought processes. See, feel, sense, or know what location you wish to interact from and then see what information comes to your awareness.

◊ On your journey, you will ask for clarification from Spirit and any spirit helpers if you need it. You might engage in what's called "a dialogue," and I will give you instructions for that shortly.

◊ If at some point in the journey you sense your physiology or energy field needs to correct itself so you can achieve the outcome you wish for, you will ask it to do so.

◊ After you do your work, before you end your meditation, you will express gratitude for the help of Spirit and any spiritual allies you have called upon. Again, the point is to foster an environment of respect and appreciation. It's important to recognize that you need and want help from powers outside yourself. Gratitude is your way of ensuring that the help keeps coming.

◊ When you end your visualization, you will see yourself returning to your body, to your heart space, and then to your mind's awareness. You will tell yourself to come back to the time and place from which you started.

◊ When back in the literal world, you will commit to following through on new behavior or ways of being or thoughts. Keeping a journal is a good way to revisit what you experienced. (Later in the book, you will learn how to perform rituals to facilitate any changes you wish to make in your everyday life, but it's good to start with visualizations that can help you gain valuable insights into your health challenges.)

The following journey illustrates the practice I taught the young woman with the back pain. It is one of many journeys in this book. It will introduce you to how a journeying process might go forward. It will allow you to practice using your mind's eye to set up an energetic environment. Finally, it will teach you a fundamental practice that can shift the unconscious paradigms within which you are working. Shifting these paradigms, or "rules," is a foundational step in charting a new path in your life. If you are not willing to release how the whole of you has been operating, you will not be able to step fully into a new way of being. The process used in the following meditation or journey is adapted from training offered by the Four Winds Society.

Carl Greer, Ph.D., Psy.D., a Jungian analyst and shamanic practitioner, uses a style of interaction within the journey that he describes as "dialoguing," which can help you gain more insights from a journeying experience. In the journey as written, you might find that the hall and any spirit guides or helpers that are with you do not want you to change your contract right now. If that happens, you will dialogue (have a conversation) with them to learn why and negotiate to gain their cooperation.

As part of the dialogue, you can ask for clarification of any messages you receive. You can learn more about Dr. Greer's ways of using a dialoguing process, and why he finds releasing something and bringing in something to be an important part of practicing *ayni,* in his books, such as *Change Your Story, Change Your Life.*[12]

Meditation
Change the Rules—
Journey to the Hall of Contracts

Before you begin this journey, come to your sacred place and enter a relaxed state. Take a few moments to reflect on some of the rules you operate under. For example, you may always say to yourself, *I always have a bad back* or *I am no good in relationship.* Or perhaps you always go to bat for your siblings in confrontations with your parents or others, saying to yourself, *It is my job to watch out for them.*

In other words, you have assumed some rules for your life, or "contracts," under which you are operating, and you have reached the place in your life where these rules are limiting your life experience, holding you back from choosing other ways of being.

For the most part, these rules can be changed, as you will see with this sacred visualization. Later, you can apply this practice to a particular health challenge and do this journey to shift the trajectory of that challenge, but, for now, choose something clear to you and easy to acknowledge. Look for some situation in which you say (to yourself), *I always . . .* or *I should . . .* or *I have to . . .* or *I never . . .* or *It's my job.*

You may want to prerecord the journey in your own voice, making sure to leave pauses in places where you will want to spend more time visualizing. In this way, playing the recording back to yourself can be a good way to allow yourself to relax more fully into the meditation.

[Begin recording]

- Prepare to journey by being in your sacred place and entering a meditative state. Use deep, slow breaths to assist you in becoming more and more relaxed. Sometimes, you can quiet yourself by breathing in a 4-4-4-4 pattern such as this: Inhale for 4 counts, hold the breath for 4 counts, exhale for 4 counts, and hold for 4 counts before inhaling again. You might want to cue yourself to move into a trancelike state the way shamans do, with a rattle or drum.

- Next, move your awareness (see it, feel it, or know it) from your head slowly down to your heart space, left of center in your chest. Feel yourself sitting in this most holy place, your heart space. Continue slow, deep, relaxed breathing.

[Pause]

- When you are relaxed and ready to move forward, ask for your guides or helpers to come join you in your heart space. See them, feel them, or know they are present. Thank them for coming to help.

- Now see yourself gently leaving your physical body and walking out onto a big field. Feel the air around you; feel the land beneath your feet. Look around this meadow, and see a big castle in the distance. You sense something of value is waiting for you in the castle, so with your helpers by your side you begin to walk toward the castle.

- See the doorway through which you enter the castle. Feel the texture of the entrance, and find yourself guided forward.

[Short pause]

- Ahead of you are many rooms and passageways, but you are drawn toward a large hall in the center of the castle. This hall is big, with golden and bright white light all around. The hall is quiet, but you can feel the high vibrational energy here. This is the Hall of Contracts. Here are stored all the contracts made by all souls as they enter a new life. Feel the holy energy here, and greet any holy beings that come forward.

[Pause]

- You see a long wooden table in the center of the hall. You walk to the table and take a seat. Magically, the current contract under which your soul is operating comes forward, the contract that you have chosen to shift today. Perhaps it appears as an open book, perhaps as a scroll that you then unfurl. You can read here the rules under which you currently operate, the rules that are guiding your life. This is your current contract.

[Pause]

- As you reflect on the contract that exists, you are reminded that you do not want to work under these rules anymore. You say to any holy beings that are present, to your guides or helpers, and to the sacred energy of the hall that you want to change the rules. You say that this contract is weighing you down, and that it is hurting your physical health (if it is), so you would like to adjust the terms of the contract. Wait to see if the holy beings agree to your request to amend the contract.

[Pause]

- If you do not get agreement, do not get upset; instead, take a few moments to have a dialogue with the sacred hall and its beings. Ask if there is something you can do to allow a change in your contract to occur. Perhaps the beings need to see a commitment from you to operate life in a different way. Have a back-and-forth conversation or dialogue, and come to an agreement.

[Pause]

- If they still do not want you to change the contract at this time, get some information as to why, and make it clear that you will be coming back another day to discuss the request.

- If this time is appropriate to move forward, and your beings have agreed, now see yourself writing your new contract on a piece of paper or parchment that is on the table. Perhaps your new contract reads "I agree to do my best to [insert the specifics for yourself] while staying in healthy balance between myself and others" or "I help others without taking on more than my share."

[Pause]

- Ask the beings and guardian spirits all around you to help you incorporate this new contract into your being and to fully remove the old contract. Allow time to integrate your new contract into yourself, into your energy field. See the old contract being filed away in the Inactive Section of the Great Hall. Now offer gratitude to the beings that have helped today.

> - You then leave the hall, exit the castle, and walk back into the meadow where you began. Find yourself returning to your body, to your heart space, and to the current time and place where you are physically present. Offer gratitude to the guides that accompanied you. And now, end your meditative journey.
>
> *[End recording]*

After completing your meditation journey, write your new contract on a piece of paper. Hang up the new contract where you can see it often. For example, you might rewrite it on beautiful paper and make drawings around the words to seal in the importance of this new deal.

Throughout this book, you will be using visualizations and meditative processes to bring forth changes in your body, mind, and spirit. Again, as many teachers make clear, your thoughts control your reality. In the next chapters, I will call upon you to use the power of your thoughts to work the practices, shift your trajectory, and see yourself as changed. In fact, this book is all about you taking the power to change your life.

Let's move ahead now to describe how I see the most powerful of medicine possible—a blend of Western medicine, which you've now learned a little about, with shamanic and even energy medicine approaches.

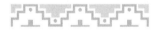

Layer upon Layer, the Power Builds
The Chacana and the Medicine Wheels

Working with the unconscious, as I learned to do and began integrating into my Western medical practice, can help you achieve changes in your circumstances. I believe in bringing back the mystical in the ways I have described. Shamanic and energy medicine enhance our abilities to achieve healing and improvements in all areas of our lives.

I've shared with you some of the intuitive experiences I've had during my shamanic training and working with clients. I've also introduced you to the basics of interacting with the unseen world to bring about change. Now I want to go deeper into the intuitive knowledge and skills I've developed.

I would like you to both better understand how I work and start to use some of my tools for recognizing your own challenges and seeing where you are on a healing journey. The mind–body connection is powerful, and while we may not be aware of programs running in the background of our awareness, unconscious rules and beliefs can strongly affect us. My hope is that by working with the tools in this chapter and the next, you can better recognize what you would like to address in your life using shamanic and energy medicine.

I began my work as a physician holding a Western medical view, namely a black or white, flat, linear view of disease (present or not present?) and prescribed medicine (working or not working?). But as I combined my training in shamanic and energy medicine with my training in traditional Western medicine, I increasingly found my assessments and prescriptions to have more power, in distinct contrast with how I had worked in the past. I began to use new ways of seeing, applying new awareness to each encounter. And I began to hold an image of each patient in a new light—on a stairstep journey that moved in a spiral, ever rising toward a peak or culmination.

When I first saw the Chacana symbol, which is integral in the Andean culture, I was transfixed. I was sitting with my sacred medicine bundle, or *mesa*, which I had assembled as part of my shamanic training in Peru. and looking at the different symbols the Quero Indians had woven into the textile. The symbol of the Chacana is representative of the celestial star formation, found in the Milky Way, and known as the Southern Cross. I have since learned that the Southern Cross is a grouping of four stars—Acrux, Mimosa, Imai, and Ginan—which can be seen as forming the shape of a kite or cross. However, even before I knew which stars comprised the Southern Cross, I intuited that the Chacana had great power.

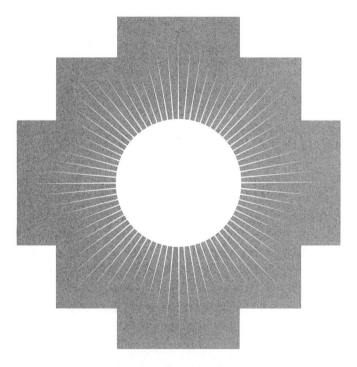

The Chacana Symbol

I could envision our human experience as being like a journey through the Chacana. You begin with an upward climb, represented by the stairs. During this climb, you gain traction on an issue as you learn and develop new skills, then you come to a plateau of sorts, where you consolidate and integrate new beliefs and habits. After that comes the next upward stairstep, followed again by the plateau of integration.

The stairsteps do not terminate at an apex; rather, they move in a clockwise fashion back to the beginning, where you once again find yourself at what some would call the beginning of a learning curve—perhaps a new challenge. You are farther along than you were before, but you must once again open to new ideas and ways. Fortunately, you have gained wisdom and developed resilience because of your journey so far. You start climbing again. And around and around the journey goes.

True to my shamanic teachings, I see a patient's path to healing moving in a clockwise manner. In the Q'ero/Peruvian shamanic tradition I was trained in, clockwise is the direction we walk around the fire and the direction we move our hands in when we wave them over a client's body as we seal their energy centers. Those are just two examples of how clockwise is considered a positive, beneficial direction. When I visualize a patient's trajectory, I see the movement—their health and life journey—as a spiral staircase on which they walk clockwise as they ascend it. There are landings where they can take a break, but the climb, the striving for something better, will never end. Maybe you can see your life as being like a climb up the spiral staircase of the Chacana?

Five Medicine Wheels

The beautiful sacred symbol called the Chacana is not the only shape I intuit when working with a patient. I also intuit five medicine (healing) wheels that give me more information about what this individual is experiencing and where they are on their journey:

1. The Medicine Wheel of the Four Directions
2. The Medicine Wheel of the Four Elements
3. The Medicine Wheel of the Four Perspectives
4. The Medicine Wheel of the Four Inner Tasks
5. The Medicine Wheel of the Four Inner Actions

Note: Even if I am not seeing patients on a given day, I bring into my awareness the Medicine Wheel of the Four Directions and the Medicine Wheel of the Four Elements. When I do so, my awareness shifts to consider the intuitive, unseen realms, so I put on my shaman "hat" when I am thinking about these two wheels.

Each of these medicine wheels has four quadrants, which, combined, represent a journey that involves challenges, plateaus, and more challenges, before you once again arrive back at the beginning—facing a completely new challenge.

Let's look at these wheels and what each represents so that you can get a sense of how they work together and begin using them to achieve greater insights into yourself and your circumstances. I'll start with the first three and leave the Wheels of the Four Inner Tasks and Actions for the next chapter, because those last two wheels are very closely related.

The Medicine Wheel of the Four Directions

The Four Directions (South, West, North, East) are most often associated with the medicine wheels of the indigenous peoples of the Americas; however, the sacred Four Directions are also part of European spiritual traditions, such as those of the Celtic people, as well as the traditions of indigenous people elsewhere.

Depending on the wheel and the spiritual tradition of which it is a part, the four compass directions can represent four steps on a journey of life (Birth, Youth, Elder, Death) or four seasons (Summer, Fall, Winter, Spring). The compass directions also are associated with four perspectives from which a situation can be viewed (Literal, Emotional, Spiritual, Energetic), and these directions are conceptually linked to four natural elements (Fire, Water, Earth, Air).

Some indigenous cultures that use the medicine wheel assign the energy and traits of an animal to each of the directions. I do not use the animals associated with a Four Directions medicine wheel to assess a patient; however, in my spiritual work, I connect with the energies of power animals, which are spiritual allies and want to help us, and I have cultivated relationships with them.

When I observe a patient to determine what ails them, data derived from my use of traditional Western medicine gets expanded upon when

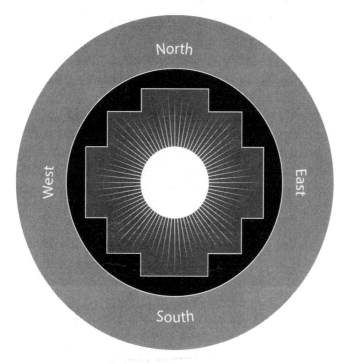

Medicine Wheel of the Four Directions

I add information from my shamanic, energetic understanding of health and well-being.

For example, as a Western physician, I might observe that a patient has pale skin, bags under the eyes, shortness of breath, and fluid in the ankles. I consider these symptoms in context of the Four Directions medicine wheel. This wheel, derived from Peruvian shamanism, has four quadrants, each of which is a point on a symbolic journey of challenges:

◊ **South** – seeing the challenge or problem.

◊ **West** – drawing upon courage to face the issue head on.

◊ **North** – taking in wisdom and understanding from ancestors or Higher Self.

◊ **East** – seeing with a new, better-educated, broader perspective because of the work in the other three quadrants.

I have taken this idea and refined it in my own way by creating the other four medicine wheels, which I use together when evaluating an individual.

When I consider where someone is on each of the wheels, I am reminded of the spiral nature and the fluidity of any situation. If we do nothing to change our circumstances, something outside of us might change them. PTSD might improve over time, when there are fewer triggers for anxiety attacks, while a health condition might worsen as the result of aging or increased exposure to toxins in the environment. At the same time, there is much we can do to improve our situation by making conscious choices that may conflict with the old rules and be in alignment with our new soul contract (if we revised ours).

Shifting any health challenge is a multi-step process. Visualizing a patient's placement on medicine wheels softens any tendency I might have to fix a physical problem in the Western medicine style and rush to get to the end of the process. My impatience is tempered, and I allow each patient the time they need for their journey. You, too, might find that by sitting and meditating with the intention of using the medicine wheels, you recognize where you are on any given wheel and what your next step in your journey should be.

The Medicine Wheel of the Four Elements

Some indigenous medicine traditions combine the Medicine Wheel of the Four Directions with the Medicine Wheel of the Four Elements. I use the wheels of the elements, perspectives, inner actions, and inner tasks together to assess a patient. In fact, I also use them with the Chacana. You might want to begin your assessment of your challenge by using the Medicine Wheel of the Four Elements, which has the following four quadrants:

◊ **Fire** – often associated with the South (picture it at the 6 o'clock position on a clockface).

◊ **Water** – often associated with the West (at the 9 o'clock position).

◊ **Earth** – often associated with the North (at the 12 o'clock position).

◊ **Air** – often associated with the East (at the 3 o'clock position).

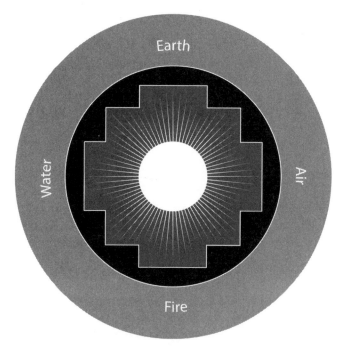

Medicine Wheel of the Four Elements

Earlier, you learned about the concept of *ayni,* or right relationship. Health and wellness involve a balance among the four elements, which are all in relationship with each other. Someone might have a lot of fluid buildup in their body (too much Water) and have a stable fluid volume but be out of breath (too little Air). Patients with joint pain and rheumatologic inflammatory conditions to me have too much Fire. A patient who struggles with behavioral issues and psychiatric complaints might lack sufficient Earth energy—their emotions are so intense that they can't focus on what's happening in their body and discuss it with me. The patient's experience of the four elements can change, so I reassess them at each appointment. (Full disclosure: My use of the elements is basic and simplistic relative to how they are understood and worked with in traditional Chinese medicine.) When working with a patient, I first sense/intuit which elements are most active and which are underrepresented.

For example, Mary is a 54-year-old woman who struggles daily with pain in her joints and mobility. Previously, I had diagnosed her with osteoarthritis, a condition where over time and with usage, the cartilage between the bones of knees, hips, and fingers becomes worn down. As it does for many, Mary's disease caused her pain and sometimes swelling in the bursa (fluid sac cushioning the joint).

When I had my Western medicine thinking cap on, the answers to her pain and lack of mobility ran this sort of course: anti-inflammatory medicine (acetaminophen, ibuprofen, or similar); glucosamine supplements (to desensitize her immune system to collagen in the hope of reducing the inflammation); X-rays (to see if her joints were so damaged that she would need a knee replacement); or referral to an orthopedic surgeon for injections (steroids, hyaluronic acid) in her knees.

Mary's lack of mobility suggested to me that she had too much Earth; her joints were stuck, as if in clay or concrete. Also, she had little motion or lift (little Water or Air). When she was experiencing inflammation, she presented with too much Fire (hot, red) and little Water (fluidity, cooling).

I would then think of ways to bring balance; for example, I would encourage her to do water exercise (increase fluidity with cooling), use a cooling liniment, take glucosamine capsules to increase flexibility, and begin a plan to bring in thoughts (Air) of healing and relieving pain into her troubled areas or simply to meditate on bringing balance to the four elements.

I told her she could sit with her journal and draw how she sees herself within the balance of the elements, perhaps something like this: her joints in the center of the page with dark brown circling them if she feels herself too Earth bound. While contemplating her "stuckness," she might then hold intentions of and draw in thoughts (Air) of healing, as if they were coming in from the outside (from the blank spaces on the sides of her drawing). In this way, she would be breathing (Air) new life into her joints, at least on paper. Mary next might draw wavy blue lines across her joints while visualizing the cooling properties and fluidity of Water.

Each thought is, by its very nature, a visualization of a beneficial change. I explained that thoughts can be brought forward into reality by drawings. If she were to combine all four elements into her drawing, she would be depicting balance among them. I explained that imagining is a powerful tool in and of itself. As we will see in later chapters, your thoughts really do steer your physicality.

I learned the most about the elements when I was working in a spiritual workshop with a group of like-minded women. My teachers (and master energy healers) CC Treadway and Lizzie Rose had us do the following exercise. I found it so powerful that to this day, the elements are an integral part of my consciousness. I hope you'll give it a try.

✿

Exercise
Engaging with the Elements

- Sit with notebook and pen, as well as drawing paper and crayons or colored paper. Engaging your full mind by writing and drawing makes for a more powerful experience. If you are not a very good artist, it doesn't matter. At the very least, feel each element, and take notes of your sensing.

- Go through the elements, one by one, starting with whichever one you sense is the right one to focus on initially. Write down all the things, positive and negative, that the element represents to you. Only after you have exhausted all your own thoughts should you consider doing an internet search of what others have associated with an element, then draw each element using crayons or markers, intuitively choosing the colors.

- Afterward, look at your picture, and consider the colors you chose to symbolize the element. Why did you choose them? Look at the shapes you drew—the specific images—and their relationship to each other. Do you see a significance to the shapes and their placement? Perhaps you drew Fire and sensed its power to burn away what is no longer serving you (for example, a "rule" that you are "always" supposed to take care of your siblings). You might then "see" yourself as the phoenix rising from the flames, unencumbered by previous beliefs.

- Finally, write a poem to each element. Your poem can be a traditional one that rhymes, a Japanese haiku (three lines with five syllables in the first line, seven in the second, and five in the third), or even improvisational jazz poetry. The point is to have fun. No rules, just your thoughts and feelings coming forward.

When I connected most deeply with the elements, I was in a group with other spiritual seekers. You may ask a friend to do the exercise with you to gain the power of two (or more) consciousnesses working on a task. Make a good-faith effort connecting to the elements before reading what I share of my sense of, and the poem I wrote to, each element:

Fire

Illuminate, challenge, transform, destroy, power, rapid, enervate, expanse, warm, dry, red

Fire – I love your heat, how you stir me inside
And the only thing possible is movement, lots of it.
You sear a trail though the underbrush
And I rejoice when we are on the other side.
If things get charred along the way, so be it.
I stripe my cheeks with the soot, my war paint.
And if all that is left is ashes
I dance in the soft cushioning under my feet.

Water

Fluid, persuasive, changeable, thunder, cold, wet, blue

Water – you cool my burning
Ah, the cool-down when it's too smoky hot.
I float inside you, and you in me.
Untethered, unburdened, we bounce
Over any rocky terrain, seeing new shores.
I dip my face and wipe the slashes of soot,
Taking time to rest along the bank
Listening to your murmurs
That sing me to sleep.

Earth

Cold, dry, solid, safe, held, supported, green

Earth – there is no liftoff
And I like it that way.
Your grasses stroke me
And your clay dances beneath my feet.
Your mud oozes between my fingers
And in it I find the alpha and the omega.
In you am I and everything else.
The primordial, the cradle, the casket.

Air

Lift, speed, stroke, swirl, power, delicate, yellow

Air – your songs pierce my quiet.
A note here, percussion there.
Flashes and flits of imagination
You speak to me in bits and verses
That broaden my horizon.
With you there is no direction –
We need no compass
To find the limitless sky.

When working with the wheel of the elements to better understand a physical or emotional ailment you're experiencing, return to these exercises you've done to see if reviewing them helps you to gain insights about your condition or situation.

The Medicine Wheel of the Four Perspectives

The third medicine wheel I use in my work is that of the Four Perspectives: literal, emotional, spiritual, and energetic.

The *literal* perspective views an issue exactly as it exists in the physical world. A patient who comes in hoping I will write a prescription to cure a health problem would be taking a literal perspective. If I begin to ask about the level of stress in their life, this patient is likely to cut me off and say, "I don't have stress; I have pain. What can you give me for it?" I might point out that they've told me more than once that their pain is preventing them from working, and I'll ask if they're thinking they will never work again and need to be on disability, but they will resist that line of inquiry, too. At a literal level, the patient sees their situation as simple, tangible, and solid: "I have a problem. I need it fixed."

At the second point on the Medicine Wheel of the Four Perspectives is the *emotional* perspective. How does the individual feel about their ailment or illness? What emotions does it bring up for them? How do they feel about their pain and the lack of mobility it has created? Is there anger, worry, resignation, or maybe even a measure of acceptance of the situation? The patient might be willing to talk about their frustration and fears about becoming dependent on their adult children. I can begin to talk with them about what's going on in their life and help them see the role that their back pain or broken ankle is playing in it.

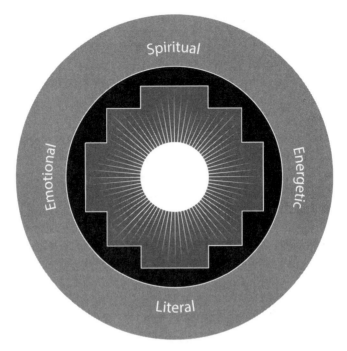

Medicine Wheel of the Four Perspectives

The emotional perspective views an issue from the place of thoughts and meanings. An arthritic vertebrae or broken ankle now is more than a weakness or break in the bone; it might represent a loss of mobility, which saddens the patient. They might be frustrated at having to depend on someone to drive them around.

I ask myself, *Is the patient receiving a payoff to being in pain and lacking mobility?* For example, does it result in more attention from their adult children? I am not a psychologist, but when I sense that someone's on the second point (9 o'clock position) on the medicine wheel of perspectives, I will guide them to talk to me about how they are coping with the emotions of their lives so I can gain some understanding of their relationships and their comfort in their lives. I will listen attentively, knowing that their health and emotional issues aren't occurring in a vacuum. While Western medicine taught me to focus on the patient sitting in front of me, I know that a patient's connection to family, friends, and neighbors can affect and reflect their health challenges. Guiding my patient to take an emotional perspective gets them to begin thinking about their thoughts and what their health problem means for them.

When someone takes a *spiritual* perspective (the third position on the wheel), they can view any issue they are having as part of a sacred, mythic journey. For example, they might see their broken ankle as a sign that they need to lay low and take a restful break from the stressors of their life—or as a sign that they need to pause to consider what they are missing socially and how they can remedy their loneliness.

I might encounter resistance from my patient when asking, "Can you see any benefit to having a broken ankle right now?" if they become irritated and say, "What are you talking about? Do you think I wanted to be off work for six weeks after so much stress?" or "Are you kidding me? It's terrible that my daughter has to take time off from her busy life to drive me to my appointments!" When this happens, I can try to nudge them toward taking a spiritual perspective. I know that can help them start to deal with issues in their lives that they have ignored, but they are not always ready to move to the third position on the wheel of perspectives.

Let's suppose you struggle with lower back pain that limits your ability to do a lot of tasks. You say you want your back pain to go away. Now let's get brutally honest with yourself. Because of your lower back pain and your limits, your husband carries all the groceries in from the car. Your daughter does the vacuuming and mopping. Truth is, you don't like doing housework. People at work jump in to help whenever the office must take all the mail and packages to the post office. You feel special and protected when others take over. When your back is acting up, your daughter offers to rub a liniment on it; the attention feels good. Are you ready to be independent again? Are you ready to relinquish all the caretaking you receive from others? Are you ready to participate in all activities, including the chores around the house?

You might need to return to full activity gradually so you can get used to being a full participant again. Maybe you can find new ways to feel connected and cared for rather than through maintaining your dependence on others. Your lower back pain might be an invitation to do the spiritual work of accepting your interdependence with other people and participating with full willingness in the give-and-take of relationships as you practice *ayni*; that is, right relationship, or reciprocity.

The fourth position on the wheel, the *energetic* perspective, is associated with stepping out of the world of matter and viewing your issue and, in fact, every issue, from the standpoint of energy. When you're adopting this perspective, you turn over all health challenges to the realm of

Spirit and the Universal Field, allowing worldly concerns to fall away. In essence, you're surrendering. This doesn't mean you don't work toward at least maintaining your current state, and even improving it, if possible. It means that you're not in denial of your challenge and any emotional or energetic influences on it. It means you're surrendering to your Higher Power and giving up your ego's need to have total control over your life.

We can't always know why our medical problem persists, even if we do everything to reclaim our previous state, from eating more healthfully to undergoing medical treatment to doing shamanic practices to release ourselves from old stories and any energies that are influencing our health. The energetic perspective is about releasing situations to your Higher Self, your spirit helpers, or the Divine (whichever feels best to you)—the ultimate in turning it over to someone else to handle.

Taking an energetic perspective means being willing to merge into the Field of Unity, where all is interconnected, trusting in our Higher Power to do what's best for us on a soul level. One of the outcomes of this belief—that we are part of the Universal Field—is that our fear of death lessens and we intuitively know our essence is eternal.

All four perspectives are valuable. I was reminded of this by one of my patients who was missing some of the earlier perspectives on this wheel and stuck in an energetic one.

Robert is a 58-year-old man who was diagnosed with prostate cancer—luckily, while the tumor was small. The day I first met him, his main question was, would I order a PET scan for him? He did not remember what the urologist had told him, although surgery was planned in two weeks. He could not tell me anything about what he had been told; all he could say was, "I don't remember."

Every question I asked him, he would say that he didn't remember. He couldn't look straight at me and looked up to the ceiling while we were having this conversation. When I suggested he call the urologist's office and ask to talk to a nurse or someone to explain things again, or perhaps make another appointment and take his wife so someone else could register what was being said, he replied, "My wife was with me at the last appointment."

I could clearly see that he was in a state of disconnect. He seemed totally unable to handle any of what was coming up for him, which is not a helpful mental state to be in when there were facts to digest and logistics to deal with in the upcoming months. Meanwhile, I had asked my nurses to hustle and call the urologist's office for records, such as the pathology report and the urologist's notes detailing the plan (radical surgery, biopsy of lymph nodes, implantation of radioactive beads), and fortunately, received the records while Robert was still present for his appointment.

As I read the reports, I asked him whether he recalled being told that the tumor was high grade on the Gleason score (he did not). The higher grade would determine whether he would have his prostate removed, radiation therapy, or medications to reduce hormonal activity.

I was wondering what he had been told. He then interrupted me and said, "I will have a radical prostatectomy in two weeks."

Red flags were now waving in my awareness. On the wheel of perspectives, he was floating in the ether—out in the space of the energetic perspective, surrendering his will and completely out of touch with the emotional perspective and only holding an overly literal perspective of "My body is broken, but the surgeon will fix me." In my opinion, to grab hold of what was required medically to save his life, he would need to get his head "in the game" and down to the literal world.

I took a chance and did something I almost never do, particularly with a new patient. I was blunt and direct and said the following to him:

> "I am going to talk to you now in a way that has nothing to do with science or medicine, but I am going to do this because I care about you and want you to come through this with flying colors. You are 'wifty,' floating off, disconnected from your life and life force. I understand that this diagnosis is overwhelming and frightening; however, to walk past this rocky road, you need to be completely present and in charge of your destiny. You have got to get a grip. You need to come down to earth, dig in, and start paying attention to all the details [*I needed him to get into the literal perspective*], so you can be in control of how your life unfolds. It is time now to get out of the clouds and be the conductor of your life. I am here any time you want to talk about how scared you are [*I wanted him to feel his emotions; that is, take an emotional perspective*], if you are sad, or if you don't understand the medical plan. For now, though, I am asking you to get your life force back in the game."

Luckily, I didn't scare him off or make him angry. In fact, his gaze became more present, and he spoke with more confidence and energy. As his appointment ended, we agreed that he would call when surgery was done and schedule another time to check in and update me on his progress.

Having a new view of any situation by "seeing" it from multiple perspectives expands your understanding. Playing with the perspectives is not only illuminating but fun.

For example, consider this. When you're walking on a gravel path, you would likely experience that the ground beneath you is uneven, and if you are barefooted, you would feel that the stones are sharp and perhaps cold. The wind might be harsh against your face, and you might recognize that you are not moving as quickly as you would be if you had shoes on. None of these sensations has any deep meaning; they are just sensations that orient you as you walk on the path.

When you're seeing from a literal perspective, everything seems to be exactly as it looks. Your understanding comes only from taking in information directly from your senses. In this perspective, you have no hidden agenda and neither does anyone else.

But what would you feel emotionally? From an emotional perspective, you might say to yourself: *These stones hurt. Why didn't I wear shoes? I am miserable. When will my walk on this path be over?*

Taking a spiritual perspective, you might say to yourself: *A hard path often leads to greater rewards,* or *I've always been good at overcoming the rough patches; I always move to a higher place afterward.*

Moving into the fourth quadrant of the wheel of perspectives, the energetic perspective, you might say a brief prayer such as: *Please help me maintain a positive attitude as I continue along this path.*

Here's another example. Let's say you are in the middle of a confrontation in your work environment. The boss's voice is louder than usual, her face is red, everyone else in the room is moving back some, and the clock on the wall behind the boss's head reads 10 minutes to noon. The office refrigerator is whirring in the other room. You are simply perceiving sights and sounds, using your senses.

Again, imagine if you were to experience the situation from the other perspectives: emotional, spiritual, and energetic.

Standing and listening to your boss criticize you, using the emotional perspective, you might think: *This is so unfair. I don't deserve this. I feel so angry at this unjust accusation.*

The spiritual perspective to having your boss chew you out might be: *The boss always criticizes people when she has trouble at home; she will soon realize it's not about me. She's just working through her old stuff,* or *Is there anything in this critique that rings true to me? I can only fix what I can control. I'm always learning, and I'm open to learning from this situation.*

Adopting an energetic perspective, you might imagine your spirit helpers at your side as you continue listening to your boss vent.

Now consider a health challenge that you initially perceive from a literal viewpoint: elevated blood pressure. You notice the number and see that both the top number and the bottom number are elevated. You notice the nurse's eyes widening as she writes down the number. Once again, what you are experiencing is information coming from your senses.

Let's look now at what encompasses the emotional perspective of each of these scenarios. As the nurse writes down your blood pressure number, you might form these internal thoughts: *I can't believe my blood pressure is so high. Will I have to take medicine? I don't want to take medicine; I hate taking pills.* All these thoughts, which you might not articulate but be having deep inside, are accompanied by emotions. You worry, you feel frustration, fear, and anger—and perhaps even shame.

Moving to the spiritual perspective, you have a different experience. You might say to yourself: *Let me think about what stressors I have been under that could be affecting my blood pressure, making my "blood boil,"* or *Is my body trying to tell me something about living a more "chill" life?*

And lastly, adopting an energetic perspective, you could take a deep breath and let it out slowly, as you intend to release to Spirit your fears, frustrations, and shame and invite in Spirit's help at addressing your high blood pressure.

To learn about these perspectives more fully, you might want to enter a mindful space, remaining more alert than you would be for a deep meditation, before asking yourself the following questions (you can journal about your answers later):

◊ Literally, in the world of my senses, what am I experiencing healthwise?

◊ Emotionally and mentally, what am I experiencing with my health?

◊ Spiritually, is there a bigger perspective to this health challenge?

◊ With regard to my energy field, what do I sense healthwise?

The last question can be very closely related to the first three, so don't neglect to ask it. Tuning in to your energy field, which surrounds you and into which your body is integrated, can help you recognize physical issues and emotions you aren't aware of when you're simply thinking about a situation. It can also help you gain spiritual insights you wouldn't be able to have otherwise. When you draw your attention to your energy field, you might find the question about what you're sensing regarding your health brings answers—perhaps *I feel depleted, I am tight and not in flow,* or *I feel separate and disconnected from the world.* You might observe things that you didn't before. *I notice my husband has drawn closer to me as I face having cancer,* or *I tend to take on all the household chores,* or *There seem to be a lot of obstacles in my path*—and the latter might prompt you to question *Is Spirit asking me to walk a different way?*

You enhance your ability to take an energetic perspective by upgrading your energy field. You can do this by more immersion in nature, which will help you shift your awareness to the web of interconnection, where all things are linked and are one. You also can achieve this upgrade through meditation.

In the energetic perspective, all worries, and thoughts and feelings are surrendered to the Universal Field. Allowing yourself to release these things to the Field, Spirit, the Divine, Source, or whatever you call your higher power builds your faith and trust.

When you adopt an energetic perspective, you operate under the belief that you have Help—Help with a capital H means energies with higher capacity than you; namely, your Higher Self, angels, Nature spirits, spirit guides, or anything in the unseen world that is beneficial and supportive of you.

When you work in the energetic realm, you are acknowledging that you are part of something bigger, and that you want to be in alignment with the larger flow, as you trust this will benefit you. You might say a simple prayer such as: "Spirit, please take over. I release all my fears and negative thoughts to You."

Again, each of the perspectives has value. A hard gravelly road can motivate you to wear sturdier shoes and thus avoid injury, or to rest more and walk less. If you are seeing the visuals described in the office scenario, you should pick up on the cues that your boss is very angry, and you are probably better poised to remain calm to respond appropriately. If you're seeing the nurse's wide eyes and high numbers on your blood pressure cuff (or she tells you about your high numbers), you recognize that she's scared because you know that's what dilated pupils mean—important signs that there is something to pay attention to.

Shamans recognize that everything is integrated—our bodies, our minds, our energy fields, and the world we share with nature and all beings. As you begin thinking more holistically about your health and your life, I hope you'll find the Chacana and the wheels you've learned about so far helpful for understanding what you're going through and how you can help yourself. There are two more medicine wheels that can be your tools. You'll learn about them next.

The Medicine Wheels of Inner Actions and Inner Tasks

As I began more deeply integrating shamanic and energetic tools into my Western practice, I developed a wheel that helps me ascertain where the patient is in accomplishing the inner work they need to do to shift a health challenge and another wheel that captures how they might engage with processes necessary to bring about a shift.

I call these the Wheel of Inner Tasks and the Wheel of Inner Actions (the actions are the Four 'A's, and I've devoted a chapter to each one). While I use these two wheels in conjunction with the Chacana and the other medicine wheels you read about, the Wheel of Inner Tasks and the Wheel of Inner Actions are so closely connected that I sometimes think of them as two wheels in one.

The Medicine Wheel of Inner Actions (The Four 'A's)

The Wheel of Inner Actions includes the stages of:

◊ **Aware**

◊ **Allow**

◊ **Act**

◊ **Affirm**

Each of these will be explored in depth in Part Three of this book, which focuses on putting Maximum Medicine into action and techniques that can help you do that.

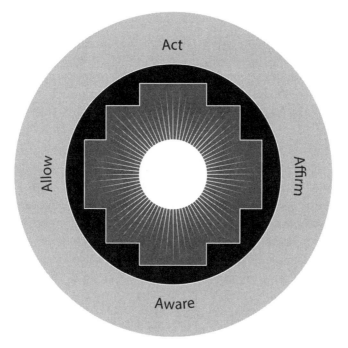

Medicine Wheel of the Four Inner Actions

I consider the following questions to determine where my patient is on this wheel and how they might progress:

Is the patient *aware* of all the issues surrounding their illness; that is, potential triggers for its onset and places where they resist a solution? A patient may be in denial or ignorant of what's going on with them aside from the most obvious problem: a symptom that's unpleasant.

Has the patient sought out help from others (*allowed* help); that is, from a confidante, a physician, or forces in the unseen world such as spirit guides, angels, power animals, and such? "Allowing" means being open to the possibilities that can arrive when you let yourself receive help from others, including forces in the spiritual world that are greater than yourself, including your Higher Self. (Your Higher Self is a part of you, but it has wisdom and understanding beyond that of your conscious self because it is in communication with Spirit.)

Is the patient ready to *act*; that is, taking steps to better their health or situation in spite of any resistance or difficulties? Have they taken action to set a clear intention regarding their healing? Do they know what they want to experience, aside from symptom relief?

Has the patient committed to *affirming* what they have learned about their ailment by applying the new knowledge and understanding to their everyday life in the long-term? The immediate action taken is important, but so is establishing new habits by setting a plan for the future.

Also part of affirming is energizing your intention; that is, following through on your goal setting and taking practical steps to change habits through ritual. I know that personal rituals and ceremonies can be very powerful tools for transformation.

The patient sitting on my examination table may be acutely aware of pain but not yet able to see beyond its existence to the possibility of less pain—or even the elimination of pain they may have suffered for years. My job is to help the patient connect with something bigger than themself, whether that be the healing power of Nature, or God, or allowing themself to have a new belief pattern that can help them to act, even to affirm, both of which are necessary for lasting change.

The Medicine Wheel of Inner Tasks

I recognize that each patient needs to undergo certain processes or inner tasks if they want to change their approach to a situation or condition. This fourth medicine wheel, like the others you learned about, has four points or steps, each of which is an inner task that can improve your ability to tackle your challenge more effectively:

◊ **Intuitive** exploration

◊ **Amplification**

◊ **Intention** setting

◊ **Ritual** (which energizes intention)

Intuitive exploration means going beyond the literal to discover what you can intuit about your situation. You need to be aware of all facets of a challenge, which requires allowing yourself to receive information that doesn't come from your analytical brain or someone else's. You must start to sense the multiple components of a health issue so that you can affect their cause. That requires getting in touch with your intuition and what you're able to feel or simply know somehow—in a way you can't explain.

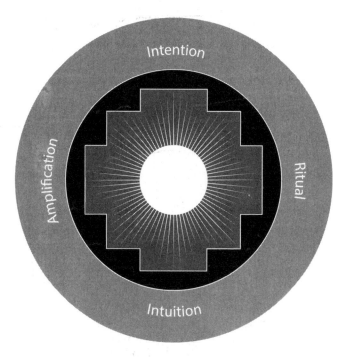

Medicine Wheel of the Four Inner Tasks

Many people are taught that intuition isn't real or trustworthy, so it often takes an internal shift to accept that it has value.

Next, you need to begin the task of *amplification,* broadening your perspective on your illness. You might consult a medical specialist, allowing that physician to give you more information that can add to your perspective, which will increase your knowledge. However, amplification as an *internal* task means going beyond your own intuitive abilities to call on allies—God, Spirit, and spirit guides such as angels or power animals—to help you have even greater intuitive understanding of the challenges before you. As you meditate or do a guided visualization (or "journey"), you'll have spiritual assistance—if you call on it. (And don't forget to reciprocate by honoring your allies and thanking them for what they do for you.)

Once you amplify your perspective, widening it, you are ready for the next internal task. If you're having a health challenge, do you want to stop feeling pain? Become more mobile? Have less pain and more mobility, so you can be more active in your community and more easily play with your grandchildren?

Set an intention for a specific, desirable outcome, but also include a grander, expanded possibility of healing beyond simply addressing a problem to make symptoms disappear. Note that doing work of the first two internal tasks helps you gain a broader, deeper perspective on your symptoms, setting you up to create an intention that is more powerful than it would be if you had skipped them. (In chapter 7, you will learn more about setting grander intentions that go beyond the limitations of the intentions you might come up with initially.)

The last internal task is to use rituals to anchor beneficial changes into the luminous energy field, energizing your intentions. While performing a ritual may seem like an external task, not an internal one, the power is not what you do and say during the ritual but the internal experience you have when you perform it. What firewood you use, how you stack it, and where you stand when you light the fire for a fire ceremony only matter if these activities have meaning for you and help you make an internal shift, energizing your commitment to seeing your intention be manifested.

For example, you might do a shamanic ritual in which you interact with a fire by sitting in a meditative, prayerful way in front of it, observing it, and then using the fire to "burn away" unwanted aspects of a health issue. You could do this by burning a stick or a piece of paper that represents that which is unwanted—a symptom, for example, or an ailment or an illness, as well as any frustrations or anxious thoughts you have as a result of the health issues. Ritual energizes you by helping you to truly feel your connection to the outcome you desire.

Let me offer an example of how the two inner wheels work together. I developed high blood pressure from stress recently. Believe me, I was fully aware of the potential consequences of leaving this untreated. I *allowed* my friend, a cardiologist, to tell me to take certain actions—get blood work done, take medications, get an echocardiogram; I didn't resist. However, I also chose to sit meditatively and talk to my spirit guide and magical helpers, asking them for help—I *allowed* that to happen, *amplifying* my personal power. I opened windows and doors to them.

My necessary act was to take the medicine, which was difficult for me as it meant admitting I needed pharmaceutical help and that my body was showing signs of aging. It meant getting past my resentment about how unfair it was for me to have this problem, but I had to take the action of following my friend's recommendations. I had to make that commitment and follow through on it with strong *intention*.

The fourth action is to *affirm*. I'd experienced an "aha" moment as the result of being aware, allowing, and acting and recognized that I had to be disciplined in establishing a new habit. Taking one immediate action wasn't going to be enough for me to reduce my blood pressure; I needed a plan for not falling back into the old ways, for getting back on the path of healthy habits if I strayed from it. I also undertook a daily *ritual* of sending my stress to the fire (as I will teach you in a later chapter).

What steps do you have to make to anchor new ways of being into your daily life? If you don't know and don't want to think about it, you're avoiding the fourth action on the wheel: *affirm*. I personally committed to a disciplined walking program and bought a fitness watch to chart my distance and time.

It is extremely difficult, and perhaps even impossible, for people to make any progress in improving a health condition if they are unwilling to consider new possibilities (*allow*) or to make any crucial changes (*act*). If there's an openness to not only allow and act but to *affirm*, to establish new habits instead of hoping for a quick fix, patients are much more likely to achieve improved health.

○

Exercise
Journaling with the Four 'A's

- A journaling exercise can help you make the most of embarking on each step of the Four 'A's. Start by making four columns or four sections on a few pages. Title each column or section *Aware, Allow, Act, Affirm*, then, in each column (section), write down everything you can think of for that stage of the wheel.

- For example, under *Aware* find a quiet place, close your eyes, and pay attention to feelings and thoughts that arise and then write everything you are aware of in the physical, the emotional, the spiritual, and the energetic realms. Add any thoughts that might float across your mind, such as "If I took a walk, I would see this challenge more clearly." Your subconscious (Higher Self) will send you messages, so take notes.

- Under *Allow*, jot down all the ways you could "allow" more. Perhaps you allow your deepest inner self to guide you, rather than the logical mind that runs your day. Perhaps you can allow/accept that sitting in meditation really does give you deeper answers. (Your note might say, "Take more time for quiet so that deeper answers can arise in my awareness.")

- Under *Act*, jot down all the ways you could act that might mean doing less, such as releasing the need to be the one with all the answers who tries to solve all their problems by themself. Often our rational mind is used to running the show; releasing its grip and acting in ways that make it easier to access our deeper parts can bring forth rich and more nuanced ideas.

- Under *Affirm*, you might note that you are willing to change your diet, spend more time outdoors, sit in sacred space, or perform a ritual to affirm your intention.

Using the Wheels of Inner Tasks and Wheels of Inner Actions Together

Although I think of them as two different wheels, as I said earlier, in some ways, the Wheel of Inner Tasks overlaps with the Wheel of Inner Actions. It may be easier for you to understand both wheels and how they interact as you read the story of Andrea.

Andrea is a 34-year-old woman recently diagnosed with a rheumatologic condition who shifted the topic of her visit with me. Her appointment started as a check-in after seeing the rheumatologist to ask for help with her mood and PTSD. I had only met Andrea three times prior to this appointment, and did not know anything about her mental state, as we were focused on addressing her severe pain and joint inflammation.

She then proceeded to tell me that when she was an emergency medical technician, she was called out to assist after a young girl had fallen off the roof and died. What Andrea remembered the most about that day was not so much the girl having died but the grandfather standing near the house, without any sense of sadness or loss and with a smirk on his face. In fact, Andrea shuddered to recall it and said that the grandfather's behavior haunts her dreams.

Instantly, I went into shaman mode and said, "You came face to face with evil." Andrea nodded her head. I clearly saw (in my mind's eye) the swirling black clouds coming out from the grandfather, touching anyone who came near enough, and that those malevolent energies had entered Andrea's field. As I always do before performing shamanic work on a client, I told her: "What I am about to say to you is not science or medicine but are my spiritual beliefs. I believe I can offer you a solution in addition to treating you medically."

So now I was totally in shaman mode. Immediately, in my awareness, I placed an energetic shield around Andrea and commanded the blackness to leave. I could easily see how the disruption to her energy field had not only led to the nightmares but also had Andrea off-kilter with depression and anxiety. Of course, when I am in a physician's office with short appointment times, doing a thorough job as a shaman is not always possible. However, I found myself setting up the energetic practice in my mind along with my intention for her field to clear.

As soon as I had said the words "face to face with evil," Andrea had nodded, wanting more. I told her that she needed to spend some time in sacred space, meaning in prayer, meditation, or simply immersed in Nature (you'll learn more about sacred space in chapters 7 and 12).

I also told her that, when in sacred space, she should call in her spirit helpers (angels, guardians, spirit guides, whatever she believed in). With a lit candle in front of her, she should use her mind—that is, her awareness, sensing, imagination, or thoughts—to pull out anything unwanted from her body, mind, spirit, or energy field that was left behind from the encounter with evil. I explained that she might sense or intuit something that didn't belong in her field as a darkness or heaviness, an obstacle, or negative energy, thought, or feeling, depending on the form it took. I asked her to practice sending the blackness out of her into the candle and ask her helpers to make sure it stayed gone. She should do this several times, and perhaps repeat the session on other days. Use of fire transforms all the excess energies; fire can be from a lit candle, a fire in the fireplace, or an outdoor campfire.

Andrea had already intuited what was wrong with her besides her rheumatism. She was aware of having been traumatized the day she found the young girl who had fallen off the roof. She understood the challenge of letting go of the energy of the memory that was affecting her. Andrea amplified the process I had begun in the office by thinking in a new way about her memory. I was glad she had allowed herself to receive help from me and would allow more to come from her spirit helpers. She was clear about what outcome she wanted—her intention—and was ready to act. I taught her a ritual to use to clear unwanted energies, and in performing it, she would be affirming her intention, energizing it.

Combining the Wheels of Inner Tasks and Inner Actions ask yourself:

◊ What do I need to be aware of? What is my intuition telling me?

◊ What do I need to allow or release to Spirit?

◊ How can I feel and then amplify a connection to Spirit and my spirit helpers so I can receive their help and insights?

◊ What action do I need to take now? What intention am I setting?

◊ What do I need to affirm through committing to a long-term plan of changing habits?

◊ How could I energize this commitment using ritual?

Combining Physiology with the Chacana

Using what I know as a physician and from my graduate training in physiology, I have been able to incorporate a sense of body systems into the Chacana. While you may not be a physician (or maybe you are!), I share this briefly with you so that you can see the possibilities of layering different approaches for a more powerful assessment of a problem. You do not have to include this awareness for yourself; just recognize that health (and life) is multifaceted. Addressing it by acknowledging and working with its many layers, using the medicine wheels you have learned about, can help you better understand and address whatever is challenging you.

I see the Chacana (each person's stairstep life journey) in the center of the wheels and align the wheels much like clockfaces, with the lowermost positions downward, at the 6 o'clock space (I'll explain more about the organ systems and the Chacana later).

At first, I only use the wheels of directions, elements, and perspectives and place them in concentric circles around the Chacana. I see each wheel spinning around a person, active at the same time. I visualize where the patient sits on the Chacana and the first three wheels; the other two wheels, the Wheels of Inner Tasks and Inner Actions, come later, when

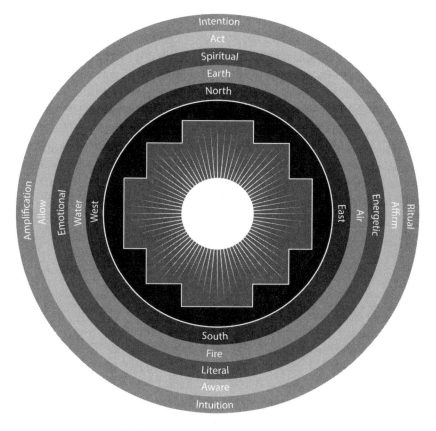

Combining the Five Medicine Wheels

I build a more complex assessment of the patient. Note that where the patient sits on each of those wheels changes, depending on the individual and the stage in which the health challenge exists.

As for you, when you look at where you are personally in each wheel, you gain a sense of the place you are in your journey, using the concepts of perspectives, directions, and elements to expand your view of yourself. You may be clear on your challenge and are building up the courage to deal with it. Hence, on the Wheel of the Four Directions, you sit in the West direction. You may be worrying and crying often, spending a lot of time in the emotional perspective. However, since beginning your inner shamanic work, you have started to dive into your physicality, emotions, and energy field. You have a clear sense that you are irritated all the time (Fire) and are stuck in your ability to make progress (Earth). You can clearly see that you are not in balance regarding the elements.

Next, you look at the Wheels of Inner Actions and Inner Tasks. You feel you are very aware but could better develop your intuition of the health challenge, and only now have you even considered allowing help from Spirit. You recognize that you need to amplify your assistance and resources. You see and know that you are not yet at the place of Act nor of setting an Intention. On these wheels, therefore, you are poised between the 6 o'clock and 9 o'clock positions.

There are two other important points. First, when you see your inner journey as a wheel, and consider where you might be on that journey, you look around the wheel and start to see a bigger picture of your health issue. You now are gaining broader vision, which is healing in and of itself. You are an observer looking at all facets, rather than feeling overwhelmed by a health situation that's out of your control. You're able to see it from a higher vantage point, which is the place where Spirit resides.

Second, it doesn't matter where you sit on any of the wheels, even if you're in the first quadrant on any of them. What matters is that you start to move, to take a journey, to flow with the river of life. You can see farther along the wheel what your journey will be and know that you have capacity to shift, transform, grow, and change. You are not stuck because of this health issue; you are looking forward. That act of looking shifts your thoughts and shifts your energy field, providing momentum for change. In future chapters, you will learn specifics about the steps along the Wheels of Inner Actions and Inner Tasks.

Now, let's bring the Chacana in. I see the wheels surrounding the Chacana concentrically. My scientific medicine brain began to "see" how each organ or system—cardiology (heart), pulmonology (lungs), neurology (nerves, spine, and brain), nephrology (kidney)—occupied a place within this layout of the wheels and the Chacana. Organ systems change, so the characteristics that are most evident one day may not be those showing another day, so how I would mentally place organ systems relative to the wheels (specifically the perspectives, elements, and directions) is a snapshot in time. With these caveats, here are some examples.

The heart is intimately associated with blood, and blood is composed of iron, and iron is of the earth; thus, I could see the heart as an Earth element. Very often, heart disease (blockage of blood vessels) has a genetic influence; thus, I might also think of the heart as being in the North with the energy of the Ancestors. Often, overcoming heart disease requires taking a spiritual approach—clearing genetic and family imprints from our

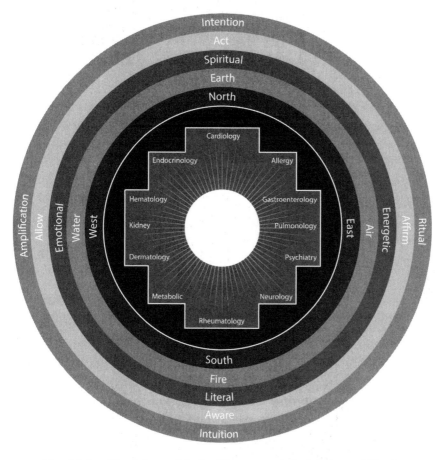

Combining Physiology with the Chacana and the Medicine Wheels

energy field and bringing in a better balance of love to our behaviors. As you think about your own health issues, do you see any of them as related to blood and the earth? Or to genetic legacies?

A second example is that of dermatology. Skin diseases can be inflamed (Fire) and sometimes blistered (Water). A skin disease can be itchy or is disfiguring, so the patient is likely to be in the literal (South) and emotional (West) realms on the Wheel of the Four Directions, experiencing physical discomfort, fear or embarrassment. These patients often are just beginning to recognize what the health challenge is. A challenge in treating a skin disease could be to cool the Fire (inflammation) and to remind the patient that they are more than "skin deep" (meaning the patient needs to see their situation from a higher vantage point, as more than their skin, so it would be good if they could shift to a spiritual perspective from an emotional and literal one).

Again, tackling a health challenge is a dynamic process. Where your health challenge might "sit" on each of the wheels is not going to be the same over time. Lung disease can easily be seen as sitting where Air is positioned. Kidneys are positioned at Water. I can see gastroenterology as between Earth and Air: solid and gassy. And psychiatry, with its focus on thoughts, sits in the Air direction, but of course it also could be in the Emotional position or in the Spiritual, depending on what the patient is engaging with (for example, if the patient is experiencing anxiety and uncertainty about their life's purpose). Which wheel you elect to relate a health challenge to, and what aspect of that health challenge you focus on, is completely your decision.

Consider for yourself the following questions and remember, there are no right answers:

◊ On each wheel, in what position does the current state of your health challenge sit?

◊ When your health issue improves, where does it reside? Is this position different from where it resides most of the time?

◊ When your health issue is more problematic (you're experiencing worse symptoms, you're more worried about it, it's interfering more with your life, and so on), where does it reside on the wheels?

When you tackle your personal health challenge, I suggest starting with the first three wheels. The Chacana is available if you wish to gain a more nuanced and complex awareness, but using it is not necessary for shifting a health problem. After you assess yourself using the first three wheels, then you can determine where you are on the Wheels of Inner Tasks and Inner Actions.

The first three wheels help you expand and deepen your understanding of your health issue. This deeper understanding is very valuable. What is needed now is to move along your journey toward wellness, so the next things to learn are the tools to make shifts. The following chapters will show you, step by step, how to engage with inner actions and inner tasks. With the important background under your belt, you can now start to be the shaman in charge of your healing.

Consciousness, Character, and Connecting to Spirit

As you will come to see, and hopefully believe, you have more power to heal yourself than you might have realized. Your awareness of your energy field, your ability to communicate with this field, your capacity (and willingness) to link to Spirit, and your fierce intention can shift you when you are stuck, even at the densest places in your energy field. Many spiritual teachers have taught that your thoughts, especially your directed thoughts, govern the destiny ahead as you exercise your healing abilities.

What does this mean? It means that you – and you alone – are responsible for every circumstance and every event you encounter in your life, and that every person you encounter can only act the way you perceive them to be.

In other words, your expectation of who they are causes them to act the way they do around you. If you think and believe a person is nasty and miserable, then that is how they are likely to act toward you. On the other hand, if you think and believe a person to be lovely and charming, then that is the way they are likely to act toward you. Your perception of them will determine what you will see.

As Rita Faith and Neville Goddard wrote in their book *Master Your Inner Game to Achieve Your Desire: Book 1, Inner Talking,* "The whole vast world is only yourself pushed out"; that is, projected onto others like a movie onto a screen. They also say, "The only way you can change your outer world is to learn and master your inner game. When you change your inner state, your outer world will and must follow it." This, they write, is a universal law.[13]

Let's start with your energy field.

As taught by many of those who work with energy—teachers such as Carlos Castaneda, Alberto Villoldo, Carl Greer, Barbara Brennan, Sandra Ingerman, and Donna Eden—each person has a luminous energy field.

This field is egg-shaped and surrounds the physical body. The individual energy field borders and merges with the Universal Field and with the fields that each object occupies, whether plant, animal, or mineral. In turn, the flow of energy from our personal field directly communicates with our physical form. Barbara Brennan's book *Hands of Light* has many good illustrations of the energy field that you might find helpful.[14]

Every experience we have had, emotional or otherwise, leaves a mark (imprint) on our energy field. Shamans work with the field to address these imprints, which influence our physical and emotional health and well-being.

As healers directing energy, shamans recognize that refined, light, higher frequencies occupy the more spiritual, etheric realms, while heavier, denser frequencies are found in the realms of matter, of physicality. The Q'ero Indians of Peru call these frequencies Sami and Hucha, respectively. (Vibration is the movement of particles, while frequency is the speed of the vibration.)

By the very nature of materiality, it takes condensing vibrations (moving electrons closer and closer together) to occupy the human form on Earth—we are not Spirit; we are matter. Some disease states, in which the physical form is stagnant, may require bringing in higher, lighter frequencies, or Sami, while other states, such as a psychiatric disconnect, may need denser, grounding energies, or Hucha.

How do we shift the flow of energy within our field to influence our physical form? By working with our consciousness—our awareness—and our command of our internal and external environments. Our awareness expresses itself in thought, and thoughts have been shown to change physical reality.

As Dawson Church writes in *Mind to Matter: The Astonishing Science of How Your Brain Creates Reality:* "Matter is not an abstract metaphysical proposition. It is a physical fact, as material as the bodies we live in. Thought by thought, moment by moment, our minds are creating the energy field in which our cells reproduce. Positive thoughts provide our cells with an energy culture in which they thrive."[15]

When you begin self-healing, an understanding of your consciousness and intention is critical. Thoughts can be more uplifting and Spirit-like, or they can be negative and exemplify the worst of human behavior. When you shift your thoughts from those of negative, lower vibrational quality to those of higher vibrational quality, you are opening your energy field to higher energies that are beneficial, allowing them to flood your personal field and affect its imprints.

David Hawkins, M.D., Ph.D., spent a large part of his life's work categorizing the vibrational differences in our inner thoughts, which he called the Map of Consciousness. As Hawkins writes in *The Map of Consciousness Explained: A Proven Energy Scale to Actualize Your Ultimate Potential*, lower-level thoughts include ones characterized by shame, greed, fear, and anger, while higher level ones have qualities such as courage, acceptance, love, ecstasy, and peace. More life energy is associated with the higher levels of consciousness, and it has been shown that thoughts coming from a higher-level consciousness by their very nature bring about higher-level healing.[16]

Edgar Cayce, a remarkable seer and healer, taught that "your mind is the builder"—that having a clear, strong, visionary mind is important for achieving the outcomes you desire. As shown in *The Map of Consciousness*, when you embody thoughts of a high vibrational level, you are embodying energies closer to that of Spirit—less dense, with more Sami. I encourage you to recognize and work with these states of being so you can affect physical reality.

The aspects of one's psyche and one's relationship to Spirit (the Divine, God, Nature) are critical to developing mastery over your health. The more you flood your personal field with elevated thoughts, such as love, gratitude, and peace, the more you align your field with the life force of the Universal Field, and the life force brings about healing.

As you can imagine, more life force flowing through you means your cellular machinery operates closer to the way it was designed: smoothly, error free, without hesitation, and optimally. Although I am not a Reiki practitioner, I can see that Reiki practices aim to attune the client's field to that of the life force within the Universal Field.

As noted in an earlier chapter, Frank Fools Crow, an Oglala Lakota healer beyond compare, described himself as a "hollow bone," which I interpret as having no human limitations to the energies moving through him that he directs to bring about healing. I imagine that he allowed high-level spiritual frequencies to come into his field and then into the client. His healings were miraculous, which to me means that he was masterful at removing any human barriers and filters that might block or negatively affect the energies coming through him. Life force flowed through him and into the client.

Given how energy works, if you want your personal field to more effectively bring in life force so that you can experience its healing, high-vibratory energy, you should begin to assess and improve your thinking and ways of mental being. It is important to try to think thoughts that have a high vibration. A thought field of high integrity, purpose, and intention will then flood your luminous energy field, which then informs your body's cellular mechanisms.

I have developed a 3-by-3 matrix of mind qualities to improve so that you will have greater power in tackling any health (or life) challenge. Similar to *The Four Agreements,* Don Miguel Ruiz's book of Toltec Wisdom, my Maximum Medicine Mindfulness Matrix illustrates areas in which to guide your thoughts.[17] I have identified nine key states of mental being and characteristics to embody:

1. Vision
2. Intention
3. Communication
4. Clarity
5. Expansion
6. Excellence
7. Wisdom
8. Power
9. Transformation

Vision

Amplifying your perspective, seeing beyond your usual windows. Traveling with your awareness to different realms, different destinies to gain knowlege and insight. Insight to the cellular level, knowing how to steer your biochemical processes toward health. Tapping into the celestial realms for soul guidance,

Intention

The straight arrow of your wish, pinning directly onto the target of your desire. Fueled by your life force, absent of any wishy-washy component. In the physical realm, intention sends specific signals to your body organism to move in the direction you choose. Intention's arrow is amplified by the input from the Divine.

Communication

Stating clearly your line in the sand, matching up the inside of you to what is shown to others, using your words to lead, unite and inspire. Working in concert with (talking to and listening to) the biochemistry, DNA, and components of your body. Listening to the voices of Higher Self, illumined beings, Nature forces and joining up with them.

Clarity

Crystal clear knowing, ability to discern words without error of meaning. Your energy field when light has shone on the shadows, when hidden agendas have floated to the surface. The flow of life force unimpeded through your Human organism, A view to the domains of the Divine, seeing the messages without opacity.

Expansion

The bigger You in your abilities, your energy field, your control over your destiny. A significant knowing of your life and its purpose. An organic awareness of your health, augmented in'considerable ways. An awareness of the ever-lasting part of you, the ethereal and infinity.

Excellence

The most amazing You in your creativity, your influence, your physicality. Your life force, life energy and life actions in major brilliance. Finding your capacities as downloads from spirit.

Wisdom

Operating from the pinnacle of knowledge. Making smart, informed decisions coming from a cohesive body, mind, spirit. In health, wisdom is knowing what serves you and what doesn't, how to shift even down to the molecular level. Wisdom is the angel's whispers in your ear, magnifying the accuracy of your choices.

Power

The full force of you, your soul, your essence coming forward unhampered by conditions around you. Power is magnified when your energy field isin alignment, and life force flows unimpeded. In health, a powerful life force Clears through any challenges, calling forth the deepest levels of healing. When joining up with the unseen world, power is limitless,

Transformation

Outcome of deep personal work, usually involving explofation and study in the dimensions of mind, body, and spirit. Alchemical shifts occur when alignments are made in the very nature of an organism. Metamorphosis can happen within the biologic and in the ethers, changing the trajectory of one's life.

The more your thoughts exemplify these features, the better you will be at harnessing your energy field to bring about an outcome you desire. One caveat is that exploring each of these mental realms is not something that is achieved instantly. The inner work you must do can last a lifetime.

The first characteristic is that of *Vision*. Vision means to amplify your perspective and to see beyond your usual windows. With vision, you can take your awareness to different realms and view possibilities of different destinies, thereby gaining knowledge and insight. You can envision the cellular level of your body and thus steer your biochemical processes toward health, or you can see into the celestial realm for soul guidance. You can record an imagined journey for yourself to access information about a health challenge.

Taking a journey of your imagination is a good way to expand your vision. Remember: When you do a visualization, or journey, you'll want to work within sacred space, opening and closing it, calling in and later, when your work is completed, expressing gratitude toward Spirit and your spirit helpers.

Another very important mental quality to master is that of *Intention*, to hold a purpose in your mind. When I visualize an intention as an energy, I see the straight arrow of a wish, aiming directly toward the target of the desired outcome. A good intention is one that is crystal clear, specific, and fueled by your deepest truths, and a powerful intention is one in which you have been completely honest with yourself about what you hope to achieve.

Your life force adds strength and potential to your intention. In healing, holding the thought of your most clear, precise, and accurate intention sends signals to your body, thereby steering it in the direction you wish. Linking up with Spirit amplifies the power of your intention.

Communication, when clear, concise, correct, and coherent, is essential when walking on your self-healing path. You will find yourself communicating with your subconscious, your body and energy field, your spirit helpers, and other healers. Make your statements reflect what you truly want. Mark your line in the sand for what works for you and what doesn't. Nothing robs the power from your statements like not agreeing internally with what you say externally.

And be certain to match what is inside of you to that which you show others. Choose the correct energy of your words to lead, unite, and inspire yourself, your body, and your energy field. For example, saying to yourself

"I hate this back pain. I hate my life!" has no healing power whatsoever. Despite any distress you have surrounding a health challenge, use uplifting words to inspire yourself, such as "I love my body. I steer my back toward healing."

Perhaps it feels insincere to say "I love my body" at a time when all you can feel is how your body is letting you down. If that's the case, shift your statements to something you can believe in, such as "I am grateful to my body and want only the best for it." The more you practice uplifting speech, the closer you will come to being able to express love even to the most wayward of body parts and machinery.

You also want to practice *Clarity*, a crystal-clear knowing or the ability to discern information without errors. When your energy field shows clarity, all your hidden agendas have floated to the surface. This happens because you are doing the work of being true inside and out and living from the higher vibrations. When you have clarity, you easily view the domains of the Divine and receive messages without opacity. For example, an inner voice might whisper to you to back off on eating cookies because you have a pre-diabetic condition. With clarity, that message is received easily and is not covered up by other mental distractions.

You practice clarity by spending more time in a quiet state developing inner awareness. You learn to slow down for a split second more so that you can stop and pay attention to the whispers from your Higher Self or Spirit. Practice that slowing down for a day or two. As soon as an awareness comes to you, briefly stop and consider it. Your fleeting thoughts may not be of enough interest to hold onto; however, the more you consider each thought, the more you can see how many messages you are getting every day and become better able to sort through and keep the important thoughts. I think you will discover that your connection to Spirit is already present and richer than you knew.

Another important mental quality to embody is that of *Expansion*. Start thinking of the bigger You—bigger abilities, a bigger energy field, and bigger control over your health and your destiny. With expansion, you can see your life and its purpose, as well as the everlasting part of you. Expanded thought involves allowing yourself to acknowledge that you can be more, and are more. Too often, our self-doubt limits the heights to which we soar. In your visualizations and journeys, have the courage to visualize yourself with even more health, even more life force than you may have at first imagined. Instead of saying, "I can't be this or that," start saying, "I can do this" or "I can be this." No inventor, leader, activist, entrepreneur, or athlete ever rose to the pinnacle of their field by saying, "No, I can't."

A useful exercise I share with patients is the following. Every time I sense that they are fearful of changing their situation and thus stuck in their current (poor) health status, I ask them, "Who made these rules (under which you operate)? Who says you can't have this (back pain go away, blood sugars improve) or do that (walk up the stairs without chest pain, bend over to do chores)?" Many times, patients will see that they hold themselves back and learn how constricted (not expanded) they are. The trick for me in showing patients this constriction is to inspire them, not bring about feelings of shame.

Excellence is an energetic and mental construct similar to expansion. When you have excellence, you experience and express the most amazing You, through creativity, influence, and physicality. In the state of excellence, life force, life energy, and life actions shine with brilliance. I find that the best way to achieve excellence is to be willing to expand and to have a strong link to Spirit so that you can bring forth your best capacities. Asking yourself, "Is this the best I can do?" is a simple way to encourage yourself toward excellence. If you are resisting or having a hard time doing something you know would show your excellence, this warrants a deep conversation with your subconscious/Higher Self/spirit guides to try to understand why. You can write and then record and undertake a journey to converse with your Higher Self and ask for understanding. Maybe there is one thing you can change to now be willing to step forward with more excellence.

When shifting a health challenge, you want to operate from the pinnacle of knowledge, namely from *Wisdom*. Wisdom means making smart, informed decisions that arise from a cohesive state of body, mind, and spirit. Wisdom is knowing what serves you and what does not, a knowing deep in your bones.

The best way to gain wisdom is to spend more time in conversation with Spirit. Spirit shows you things your conscious mind might not be able to access. When conversing with Spirit through meditation, you get answers. You will know these answers are correct and wise by at least one criterion: how you feel when they come to you. Truth feels right and good, in your body, in your knowing. Truth is a coherence between the emotions you're expressing and the emotions deep inside you. Whether a piece of knowledge is truthful or not is best determined by how it feels, not what you think about it. Your conscious mind (your head) can easily be fooled; your body (your heart) cannot.

In healing yourself, you also need to embody *Power*. Power is the full force of You—your soul or essence (two words to illustrate the same thing), both coming forward unhampered by conditions around you. Your personal power is magnified when your energy field is flowing with life force, and health is free-flowing, unimpeded life force.

How do you walk in your own power? How do you bring forth your hidden power? You do it by exercising *Courage*. How do you gain courage? By spending time in communication with Spirit to access your deeper self. You begin to listen to those whispers from deep within yourself. You can create a visualization to travel to the sacred space of your essence (deep inside your awareness, often seen by mystics as residing in the heart space) and have a conversation with the wishes, dreams, and desires of that essence: You. Visualization can also bring you face to face with your Higher Self or your spirit guides for dialogue to gain knowledge that can empower you.

To clarify how I see the difference, albeit very slight: Your soul is an eternal energy, conscious, part of the vast universe, and extends energetically into the cosmos. I see your Higher Self as part of your soul, as being like an angel on your shoulder—your conscience. Both your Higher Self and your soul tap into what is true in the universe and can be communicated with. Some might say that I'm splitting hairs in distinguishing between the two, but that is how I understand and experience them.

Lastly, dream of and then begin to believe in *Transformation*. You can achieve transformation through deep personal work, exploring and studying the dimensions of body, mind, and spirit. Your inner work, particularly that of connecting deeply with Spirit, will bring about alchemical shifts in the energetic configuration of your organism. This inner work creates a metamorphosis and an evolution of your health.

Fundamental Concepts and Practices
for Doing Shamanic Work for Healing

When you begin the work to shift your health challenge, there are some fundamental concepts and practices you should learn about and practice:

◊ Work within sacred space, respecting the sacredness of shamanic practice.

◊ Set and hold your intention, recognizing its power.

◊ Practice *ayni,* offering gratitude for the help you receive.

◊ Perform rituals, connecting with Spirit and the unseen world.

In other words, undertake all of these actions with reverence.

Sacred Space

While you've learned a little about sacred space and *ayni* already, it's helpful to go deeper into what they are and why acknowledging them is vitally important for the work you'll be doing.

As I said, sacred space can be a place where you do shamanic work, such as a spot in your home, in a sunny room, or in a natural area that feels powerful to you. Sacred space is also an inner space you open up so that your energies enter the realm of Spirit. In sacred space, you intend to feel your connection to Spirit and access the part of yourself that is eternal, that is one with all of creation. It is here where you join up with energies of power animals, of angels, of mythical beings, and of forces of nature to summon their ability to assist you.

Sacred space can be accessed through prayer, meditation, and being out in nature experiencing quiet time. Quiet time is not automatically sacred. After all, you can use it to consider who to vote for in the office football pool or what you should make for supper. Quiet time becomes sacred when you declare that your thoughts are now going to be from the deepest well inside yourself, when you wish for the highest outcome as a result of our work. In other words, you are setting aside any fears or doubts, trusting in Spirit, and opening yourself to possibility. In this way, the highest outcome is encouraged as you are doing the work in a sacred manner.

When beginning important mystical work, such as asking for assistance in shifting a health challenge, you should give notice when you are entering the sacred by doing an invocation or a prayer. When you are finished with your sacred work, close space by offering gratitude to the energies and field in which you spent time. You want to build a respectful relationship with Spirit and your allies and ensure their help in the future. Once sacred space is closed, you can then return to your normal day—with thoughts about football or supper or whatever you wish.

What follows is the invocation taught to me in my Four Winds training. The energetic boundaries around you—South, West, North, East, below (Earth), and above (Sky)—are established, providing protection as your energy body enters the Universal Field. Many indigenous people see Earth as feminine and Sky as masculine, complementary energies that together create balance, so the invocation includes a summons to Mother Earth and Father Sky. The archetypal energies associated with each of the power animals invoked bring primordial energies to bear during your inner work. As you engage shamanic energies more often, you may choose to open space calling forth the presence of spiritual allies, such as power animals, with whom you have cultivated relationships.

Whether you are working outdoors or indoors, you might want to move to face each direction you summon as you open sacred space and look upward as you call upon Father Sky and downward as you invite Mother Earth to assist you. I was taught to start at the South direction; however, you may choose to start with any direction. I advise you to keep the order the same each time you open space so that you build up the energy of this ritual each time you perform it. Also, after the invocation, pause to feel an energy of gratitude for the assistance that will come from Spirit. Hold onto this feeling as you do the sacred engagement with the unseen energies.

○

To the Winds of the South

Great Serpent.
Wrap your coils of light around us.
Teach us to shed the past the way you shed your skin,
To walk softly on the Earth.
Teach us the Beauty Way.

To the Winds of the West

Mother Jaguar.
Protect our medicine space.
Teach us the way of peace, to live impeccably.
Show us the way beyond death.

To the Winds of the North

Hummingbird, Grandmothers and Grandfathers, Ancient Ones.
Come and warm your hands by our fires.
Whisper to us in the wind.
We honor you who have come before us.
And you who will come after us, our children's children.

To the Winds of the East

Great Eagle, Condor.
Come to us from the place of the rising sun.
Keep us under your wing.
Show us the mountains we only dare to dream of.
Teach us to fly wing to wing with the Great Spirit.

Mother Earth

We've gathered for the healing of all of your children.
The Stone People, the Plant People.
The four-legged, the two-legged, the creepy crawlers.
The finned, the furred, and the winged ones.
All our relations.

Father Sun, Grandmother Moon, to the Star Nations

Great Spirit, you who are known by a thousand names.
And you who are the unnameable One.
Thank you for bringing us together.
And allowing us to sing the Song of Life.

❖

Remember, at the conclusion of your sacred work, it's important to close space by offering sincere gratitude to the six directions and whatever helpers you have called in. Again, you might want to move to face the South, West, North, East, Father Sky, and Mother Earth as you acknowledge and address them.

Set and Hold Your Intention

A key component to successful shamanic and energy work is intention. As I described previously, intention is a laser-focused thought on achieving your deepest desire. That thought should be true to what you really want—perhaps becoming financially secure as opposed to wildly rich, perhaps experiencing improved mobility in your joints as opposed to becoming a world-class athlete. Most of all, you need to suspend all the negative chatter in your mind when you hold the intention. As your mind is truly "the Builder," as Edgar Cayce described it, you do not want to jumble it with conflicting thoughts and self-doubt.

An intention has the power of your essence (your soul) behind it. When you formulate your intention in sacred space, the intention has your personal power, the power of your Higher Self, and the power of the Universe you have allied with. Personal power can come from simply focusing your mind; however, when you call on your Higher Self, you are accessing the eternal essence of You and thus are imbued with more power. You are engaging your human mind (personal power) and your deep spiritual nature (Higher Self).

As you are the one generating your thoughts, how you hold your wish for healing determines your success. Maintain your intention, infusing it with power, by believing wholeheartedly that the outcome is true already. When you do this, all is possible.

Lastly, saying or thinking that intention multiple times, not just when doing shamanic work within sacred space but during your everyday activities is important to achieving success. (You'll learn more about creating intentions in chapter 11.)

Practice *Ayni* and Express Gratitude

Shamans throughout the ages have understood and practiced the principle of *ayni*, which, as you learned earlier, means "right relationship." To maintain your sacred relationship with the energies of the Universe, the forces of the unseen, or the power of your allies, you need to stay in balance. Everything you receive or ask to receive should be balanced by what you give away or give back. You cannot be a taker, out of balance with being a giver; this is an unsustainable relationship with the Universe.

I also see the need for balance as an issue of respect. If you, as a shaman, call upon your unseen helpers for special favors and then walk away without offering gratitude or a gift, your helpers may choose to not answer your call the next time you seek their assistance. The best way to be sure you are practicing *ayni* and maintaining balance is to dialogue with Spirit or your spirit helpers to learn what they want from you.

Sacred dialogue, in order to gain knowledge to help yourself with a problem, most often contains these concepts: You ask the Universe, Spirit, your allies, your Higher Self, "What do I need to know to shift this issue? Can you help me? What should I do?" Once you have received the knowledge or gift these forces have bestowed on you, you then ask how you can reciprocate, saying, "What may I give you in return? What do you want from me?" In this way, you practice *ayni,* or right relationship, and are deeply respectful. Most often, when I ask what I may do in return, the answer I get is not to give back a material gift but rather to make the promise that I use my gifts to be better in the world, to act with greater balance and harmony, to promise to bring my best self forward, and to be of greater service to our web of interconnectedness.

Perform Rituals

Shamanic processes often involve rituals. Rituals energize intentions so that what we hope for can become manifested in the world. In reverently performing rituals that you have prepared for, as directed in this book, I think you will find them to be so powerful as to cause you to experience an inner shift.

The invocation for opening sacred space, the order of questions we ask of our helpers, the invitation to our allies, or the use of fire to bring us into deep focus and transformation during communication with Spirit all might be a part of a shamanic ritual.

These fundamentals underpin the techniques you will use when working to shift your health challenge. In the next chapter, we will spend some time on understanding the importance of shifting your personal story from one of illness and deficit to one of healing and possibilities.

Lose the Story, Lose the Past

Change can be scary. However, let's be totally honest. If no change occurs, your health challenge will be unaffected; you will be stuck. If you are unwilling to change, even the slightest bit, it means you are unwilling to be different: to have different (and improved) physiology and to walk on a new road, one of healing. One of the fundamentals of shamanic work is to let go of old ideas about yourself and what you can experience to make way for new beliefs.

When talking about moving forward to healing, one of the most common issues I see with my patients is stuckness. Often, people cope with their health issues by accepting the way their situation appears to them. They will often hold onto an inner story as to why they are having the experience. They tell me "I have gallbladder disease [or back pain or skin cancer or high blood pressure] because it runs in my family." Or, perhaps, "I have back pain because I have to stand on concrete floors all day at work." Or, "My mother has problems with her nerves; I get it from her."

The minute you make that sort of statement, one that is declarative and aligned with the current way in which you perceive your experience, you are putting up bars in the cage that surrounds you. Let me explain.

If you have said that the only thing you can experience is what others in your family have—your mother struggled with her nerves, your father had high blood pressure, your grandmother had gallbladder problems, and so on—you have relinquished your independence. You have defined your power as being within the limits of how things seem to operate. You are, in effect, putting yourself in a cage that limits and traps you. Your words indicate your underlying belief about your limitations, and your belief is neither expansive nor transformational.

Spiritually speaking, each of us has a luminous energy field, and we are constantly sending beams of energy (light) forward with our thoughts, even when we don't express them aloud. Our destiny flows on the current of those beams. It is as if we are shining a flashlight ahead of us, projecting forward beams of our thoughts that direct our actions, illuminate our path, and determine where we move to. Fortunately, we are not limited to traveling along the direction most beams are going.

Imagine the arc of light cast by a flashlight. The majority of the light beams aim at one spot on the ground in front of us. However, the beams spread somewhat, with some of them landing on the edges of the spot, away from the center. It is the shaman's job to work with, travel along, and help the client to shift into moving on the current of a beam along the edge. In other words, the client might be likely to develop high blood pressure, like their father had, or gallbladder problems, like their grandmother had, but there are other possibilities that might defy the odds a physician offers. The shaman can help shift a person's destiny path away from the momentum of the majority and toward the minority.

In books such as *Power of Silence: Further Lessons from Don Juan,* Carlos Castaneda wrote about human perceptions from the perspective of the energy field.[18] In essence, he said that humans have beams of light emanating from them in a ball-shaped pattern (or what some shamans describe as a luminous energy field, which, as I said, is often perceived as egg-shaped). On one point on the surface of this ball, beams congregate, extending outward to the outside world. Whatever point the beams touch and illuminate in the outer Universal Field opens like a window, lighting the way to our "seeing" whatever is being expressed in that part of the field. That slice of perception, that window, is much smaller than the totality of existence. Castaneda called this congregation of beams the "assemblage point" and said we all have one.

In other words, we perceive the part of the Universal Field that our congregated beams touch and light up. We see only that with which our outward focus interacts, but this is a limited view relative to the whole of the universe. Collectively, humans congregate their individual beams and "open" the same "window" of the Universal Field. We share a collective reality, a shared perspective.

Shamans, Castaneda explained, can shift their assemblage point, allowing them to perceive reality in different ways. By setting an intention to change the position of the assemblage point, the shaman causes an individual field to touch a different part of the Universal Field. That in turn causes a change in perception for the person the shaman is helping.

How can adjusting the assemblage point's position work for us in our journey toward health? I have talked about thoughts determining outcomes and intention shifting reality. When you approach a health challenge, be ready to think in a new way and to hold the most powerful intention. Energetically, as understood by shamans for millennia, you are aligning your energy field with a different part of the Universal Field, one that links up with your desires, with your new intentions. Consequently, you can change your perspective and thus, your reality.

Here is another way to think about your assemblage point and your perceptions. When you hold an unmovable thought ("I have back problems just as my father did"), you have linked up with the part of the Universal Field where you have back problems that are not going away. You've done this by accessing the reality that says you are just like your father and therefore have the same pains.

As I said, your assemblage point is linked up with a very limited reality. You have built a cage around you, one of thoughts that anchor you and keep you boxed in. As soon as you decide to change your thought (perhaps to "I can heal myself; I can be free of back pain"), you are linking up with a new reality. You have decided to open the door of your cage and even open a window in the metaphorical room in which you live. When you shift your thoughts, you shift your assemblage point and thus, your reality.

Now, on a day-to-day level, you probably won't be thinking of assemblage points and realities. But you should be thinking of being and living in a new world, one of new possibilities rather than one of probabilities. To do that, you must change your thoughts and, in turn, change the way in which you speak about yourself and your health and your destiny—the "story" or explanation you have for what you have experienced, are experiencing, and will most likely experience. You must be willing to have a different way of framing your past, present, and future.

Of the many challenges I face being a physician and shamanic healer (other than navigating the issues around the darn COVID-19 virus!) is helping patients change their story, their language, and their limiting beliefs. Almost daily, I have a conversation with someone in which I say, "Who says?" or "Is that a rule that can't be broken?" We then begin to talk about the cages that are built due to the patient's limiting thoughts, whether the patient can see how boxed in they are, and if the patient is willing to change. I often lead with, "What if this issue could be fixed?" or "What would it look like to be free of this issue?"

Believe it or not, not all patients want to change. They might say they do, but digging deeper, they start to see that on some level, they want their situation to remain the same. As I talked about in a previous chapter, there can be benefits to staying in a limiting position with regard to health, including getting attention from other people. That is why you must be very honest with yourself about what you gain from retaining a limitation. And, unfortunately, some patients wear their diagnoses proudly, as if they had been awarded merit badges—the badge of hypertension, the badge of chronic pain, the badge of autoimmune disease. Sometimes it feels to me as if they want to be noticed by declaring all the diagnoses they have.

If you see having a diagnosis and disease to be meritorious and validating, you will need to do some significant work to move toward a more healed state. You could start by using a fire ceremony to clear your thoughts and burn away unwanted aspects of a health issue, as described previously, and seeking guidance from an energy or shamanic worker and/ or a psychotherapist.

Often, a patient has lived so long in the story of herself with different diagnoses that it is hard for her to imagine herself without these issues. If you are asked to describe yourself to someone you are just meeting, and your description of yourself includes "I am 42 years old and suffer from a bad back and arthritis," you are declaring those items to be part of your essential existence. It is quite different to say, "I am 42 years old and am working hard on living to the fullest, physically mentally, and spiritually."

For a long time, one of my best friends would always start her conversations with why she didn't want to work anymore—because she was too old. What she meant was she had progressed far enough in her life to deserve retirement, but what she stated was that she was old. After a few years of these kinds of statements, and of me grumbling that she should stop saying those things, she developed an autoimmune disease that significantly limited her movement and functionality. She acted as if she was old and felt old.

Shifting your perception of disease and limitation so that it is a condition you are living with, not a defining issue that is core to your identity, will go a long way in helping you shift your health challenge. Luckily, with many purposeful changes in her life, my friend's autoimmune disease is in remission, and she is limber and lively. She no longer says things like, "I am too old." Choose your words carefully when you talk about your current state and your future. And remember to keep your thoughts in the realms of what I call the Maximum Medicine Mind Matrix—that is, make sure they are expanded, transformed, and powerful.

Exercise
Drawing a New "Story"

To begin engaging with the story from the past that has kept you on a certain path, try this writing and drawing exercise. You will need a large piece of paper, at least 14 by 17 inches. You also can tape a few sheets of letter-size paper together. Turn the paper so that the longer side is horizontal. Gather some colored pencils, crayons, or markers you can use for drawing.

- Next, enter sacred space. Remember to ask and allow Spirit and/or spirit helpers to assist you in this work. Set an intention for your transformation.

- When you're ready, draw a stick figure on the left third of the paper. Leave at least an inch free along the bottom of the paper. Then, draw a fire in the center of the paper—it can be a firepit, a candle with flame, or whatever else you choose to depict this element of transformation. Color your fire to show its power and beauty.

- Next, draw a stick figure on the right side of the paper. Along the bottom of the paper draw a horizontal line, which will be a timeline, and label today's date under the stick figure on the left.

- Think about all the issues challenging you from the physical, mental, or spiritual realms, and write them around the figure on the left side. This is the current you. Use color, words, and symbols to indicate the issues that are impacting you. Feel each issue as you draw or write it. For instance, if you have high blood pressure as an issue, you might write about it, placing words all around the stick figure on the left, which represents your present self, because you feel this health problem affects every part of you. You might draw your head in red, or perhaps black, when you recall the headaches you sometimes get. Surround the stick figure by drawing and/or writing about every issue distressing you right now.

- Keeping your energies in the sacred space and working from the place of your Higher Self, look at your drawing, and focus on one issue at a time. Consider how this issue has impacted you and how you would like it to change. As you think about the change you would like to experience, draw a representation of that issue moving into the fire and then being burned away and transmuted. Perhaps you will draw a line from the issue near the stick figure on the left to the fire, or perhaps you'll draw a swirl of red and black representing high blood pressure that moves into the fire. As you do this, feel the issue changing. Feel the forces of the Universe making a powerful shift.

- Next, underneath the fire, on the timeline, mark a time when you want this health issue to be gone or resolved. Two days? One month? Six weeks? Remember, you might be experiencing some benefit to having a health challenge, such as having others take care of you, validating your belief that you belong in your family because many relatives have the same challenge, and so on. You may need some time to give up that benefit and find other ways to gain assistance or validation.

- Next, to add to the energetics of transmutation, you're going to eliminate the issue on the paper. Draw or write over the issue, place a slash through it, color over it, or maybe draw a cloud around it and imagine the cloud carrying it away as it floats upward. Do this for each issue. Mark on the timeline when you expect each issue to be gone, and on your drawing, as you did before, place each issue in the fire. Be sure to feel the energy of erasing, of dissolving, of releasing. Perhaps you will draw the fire brighter and bigger as you intuit its transformative power.

- Finally, look at the stick figure on the right. This is the transformed you. Note what colors you used to draw it. How do they make you feel? Do the colors make you feel more joyful or inspired? Notice the freedom you feel in your body, mind, and spirit as you draw the improved you. Take note of how this new you appears and how you feel looking at them. Lighter, maybe?

- Pay attention to whether you bring any old issues forward into the new version of you. If you do, do not despair. You may want to repeat this exercise. Many issues are deep seated and take more awareness and intention to clear in a meaningful way, and you may need the practice of working in sacred space to evoke the most powerful shifts.

When you are finished, please be sure to offer gratitude to the energies that joined you, including your Higher Self and awareness, and to close sacred space. You may wish to post this drawing in a place where you can reflect on it. Keeping the images of the shifts in the forefront of your mind will maintain your intention and the energies you worked with.

In the next chapters, I define the discrete steps to use in your healing journey.

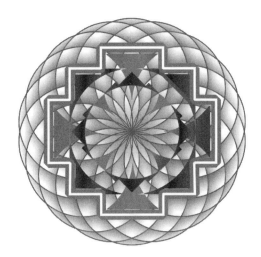

Part Three
────────

APPLYING MAXIMUM MEDICINE THROUGH THE FOUR 'A's

Maximum Medicine:
Becoming Aware

This chapter and the subsequent three chapters show you how to tackle your health challenge following the Wheel of Inner Tasks and the Wheel of Inner Actions. As I have said over and over, you may wish to embark on an inner journey of gaining more evidence to assist you in healing and shift your thinking so that you have a vision of a transformed you and hold onto it.

To take this important journey, you must devote to it much quiet time in sacred space. Please don't be daunted by the work I'm suggesting you do. The knowledge and the power over your destiny you will gain are very much worth the effort. Along the way, especially in the next chapter, you will encounter friends and companions in the spiritual realm and build a closer relationship with your Higher Self. This journey will be exciting and life affirming.

Much of this work involves intuition, which comes from listening to your inner voice, particularly when you are in concert with your Higher Self and Spirit. Intuition grows when you practice trusting that inner voice and act following the guidance. Intuition can be a knowing, a thought that appears in your mind, or a physical sensation.

My strongest intuitive signal when I was younger was a stomachache. I learned that if I was faced with a choice, and the decision I made was soon followed by a stomachache, then that choice was likely not the right one. These days I do not have to wait for a signal as uncomfortable as a stomachache; instead, I am aware of the whispers in my mind that nudge me away from bad choices and decisions that are wrong for me.

In these next four chapters, I will take you through the steps on the two wheels I mentioned. The work is broken down into steps, but you will soon see that each of these has continuity and overlap with the subsequent steps. Your mind can hold a network of information and perform many tasks concurrently. I have broken the process into small, separate bundles so that it will be more manageable. The work starts with not just understanding that you have a luminous energy body but sensing it.

Sensing Your Luminous Energy Body

As I said earlier, you have an energy field that extends outward from your body in all directions. Initially, you might not be able to sense your luminous energy field, but with practice and intention, you can. In time, you might be able to not only sense this field but also extend it outward even farther, allowing you to pick up on more information from the Universal Field that surrounds and includes all of us.

Your luminous energy field interacts with all that is around you. Have you ever felt someone behind you staring at you? You might have felt a tickling or nagging feeling at the back of your neck and turned around to see that your instincts were correct: Your field was taking in information from another's field. In fact, your field takes in enormous amounts of data that you do not consciously register or pay attention to.

If you can start to pay attention to the whispers of data, you will gain more knowledge about your environment. When you allow your sensing ability to be heard, you pay attention to the less noisy streams of data. You can do this by meditating and doing inner work. The more you quiet the loudest data streams, the more you'll start to know about the world around you. Your intuition will grow. Without changing anything in your external environment, you will now increase your awareness and ability to see and know things that are happening that your ordinary senses don't pick up on.

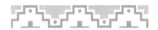

Exercise

Feeling and Working with Your Energy Field

Let's practice feeling energy with your hands. As we practice feeling energy, we are building awareness in the more subtle realms. Your hands are very sensitive, so they are a good place to start our sensing exercise with.

- Hold your arms out in front of you in a relaxed fashion. Turn your palms toward each other, and hold them 12 inches apart. Close your eyes, and see if you can sense anything between your hands. You may just feel pressure between your hands, but often it feels like a ball. Keeping your eyes closed, gently move your palms toward each other as if you were squeezing this ball. When does one hand start to feel the other? Does this occur before your hands touch?

- If you don't feel anything until your hands touch, let's shift your awareness out of your literal thinking mind and into your sensing mind. With your eyes closed, take some nice, deep breaths, in through your nose and gently out your mouth. For several breaths, follow the motion of the air as you draw it in and release it, sensing this movement with your awareness rather than your thinking. As you focus on your breath, and refocus as other thoughts come into your mind, you can move yourself into the sensing realm.

- When you are good at simply tracking your breath with your feeling, sensing mind, repeat the ball-squeezing exercise. With practice, you likely will notice that if you move your hands farther than 12 inches apart, you can still sense that there is a ball of energy between them, and that space between your hands, that ball, can get bigger and bigger, yet you still feel it. When you are able to feel energy, you are one step closer on the path of shifting energy from your field. Sensing energy is the first step toward moving energy.

- Next, let's do another sensing exercise. While sitting in a comfortable position, imagine yourself within a sacred bubble that is your light energy field. I experience this as energetic mosquito netting—woven, delicate, and vibrant. As the sacred bubble of your light energy field is at the border of your individual field, it can be impacted by foreign energies coming in and damaging the woven tapestry, so you want to repair any flaws in it.

- To begin, reach up with your hands to the space 15–20 inches above your head. The shamans of the Andes identify this space at the border of your luminous field to be the source of the sacred, the seat of the soul. The ancient medicine men and women of the Andes called it the *wiracocha* and were able to visualize streams of multicolored lights streaming from it. The multicolored streams were energy streams within a person's luminous field.

- Bring your hands down from the soul space and notice the *wiracocha*: Follow the flow of energy like water spilling in a waterfall all around you. As you bring your hands down, know that you are retracing the journey that the multicolored light filaments make as they travel from your *wiracocha* at the top of the energy fountain down and all around your body. Do you sense the energetic border of your luminous field and the movement of energy? Repeat taking your hands up to your *wiracocha* and bringing them down again to sense the light filaments that surround you. Do this until you can start to feel them.

- Now, with your eyes closed, staying in sensing mode (not thinking mode), work your hands up and down the inside of this energetic netting, or tapestry. Feel the integrity of this bubble, and notice any imperfections in it—wrinkles within the energetic fibers, for example.

- Remember, everyday interactions with the world make imprints and impacts on your energy field. As you work your hands, when you sense where the tapestry is broken, or if you sense something that doesn't belong, smooth out and repair the imperfections.

- Use your intuition to guide your hands as if smoothing spackle on dry wall or weaving new fibers into breaks in the tapestry. Work all around the inside of this bubble. To reach the part of the bubble that is behind you, use your imagination.

- The more often you work on sensing your tapestry, the more awareness and subsequent control you will have over your energy body. You can restore it in the places where it has been harmed by your experiences, and the repair work you do will, according to shamanic tradition, affect your physical body encased within the bubble.

Your intention here is important: The more you intend to repair your field, the more restoration you'll be able to do!

○

Exercise
Bringing in Earth and Sky

Here is a simple but effective way to invigorate your energy field. Invigorating your field brings in your life force, thereby strengthening your vitality. It also rejuvenates your connection to Earth and Sky, two essential partners on your spiritual and energetic journey. You can do this as often as you want. I find it to be a marvelous way to start your day. Ideally, you'll work with it outside in a park or your yard to connect to the immense field of Nature. If you are inside, imagine connecting to a natural area outdoors.

- To begin, determine the four compass directions relative to where you are standing. Start by facing South. If you are performing this exercise in the morning, you might like to face East to greet the Sun and the new day. I personally start at South, as that is the starting point for all my wheels, so it has become a habit for me.

- Extend your arms on both sides, then gently bend over and make a scooping motion with your arms, drawing in energy from the earth. Return to a standing position as you use your arms to bring that energy to your lower belly. As you continue moving them upward, to your heart, feel the energy as you're working with it.

- Next, open your arms to the sky, and scoop energy down onto the top of your head and continuing moving it, bringing it to your heart. Repeat scooping from Earth and then Sky, doing a minimum of three cycles facing each of the Four Directions.

- To make the practice more effective, inhale as you stretch to scoop and exhale as you draw the energy to your body. And while you're doing the exercise, notice how you feel. More alive? More expanded? What do you notice about your energy field?

Running the Colors

The exercise below was taught to me by C.C. Treadway. It refreshes and strengthens the light frequencies in your energy field. It will also help you maintain awareness of your energy body, increase your intuition and visualizing capabilities, and infuse your energy body with vitality, even as it repairs and restores it. Finally, using it will help you gain increased vitality and internal rebalancing, both of which are assets for shifting a health challenge.

The exercise tracks each of the colors on the visible light spectrum (red, orange, yellow, green, blue, indigo, and violet—which you can remember with the acronym ROY G. BIV). I suggest "running the colors" after you have performed the initial sensing exercise of Feeling and Working with Your Energy Field several times.

○

Exercise
Running the Colors

- Sit quietly, and close your eyes. Allow your breath to soften as you track the inbreath and the outbreath, becoming more and more relaxed.

- Holding an awareness of the energy bubble surrounding you, your light energy field, picture the color *red*—the red of a rose, an apple, or a male cardinal. See the red in your mind's eye or, if that's difficult for you, imagine it. Now, sense the red filling your field, front to back, above your head, and down to your toes, even filling the spaces between them. Sit in the energy of red as it saturates your field. Intend to rejuvenate the red filaments of light in your tapestry, then sense and visualize that happening.

- Next visualize or sense the color *orange*—the orange of a tiger lily, a calendula, or a pumpkin. Fill your field with orange, front to back, top to bottom. Sit with the orange, and restore the orange filaments of light.

- Now, move to *yellow*—the yellow of the sun, a goldfish, or the center of a daisy. Fill your field with yellow, front to back, top to bottom, all around you. Sit in that energy for a while, restoring the yellow filaments.

- Now, move to *green*—the green of a field of grass, new tree sprouts, or asparagus. Fill your field, and sit with green for a while, as you restore the green filaments.

- Next, bring in *blue*—the blue of a clear sky, a robin's egg, or the core of a flame on your stove. Fill your field, and sit in blue for a while, as you repair and revitalize the blue filaments.

- Now, fill your field with *indigo*—the color of eggplants, purple grapes, blueberries, or "red" (purple) cabbage. Saturate your field with indigo, and hold that sensation for a while, restoring the indigo filaments.

- Lastly, bring in *violet*—the color of lavender, amethyst, and hyacinth. Fill your field with violet, and sit in this energy for a while, allowing the violet filaments to be repaired and restored.

- Sit with new awareness of your energy body and its multiple frequencies of light. End the exercise when you are ready.

After you have begun to sense your energy body, bring your knowledge and understanding of it into your daily life. I suggest starting outside, in Nature. When you find a place that speaks to you, enter a state of quiet reflection, and consider the following: What drew you to this place? The scene? The colors? Is there something deeper? Can you feel a connection to the trees or the water or the rocks? If they spoke to you, what did they say? Are they saying something to you now?

If you have a hard time imagining what this natural place is communicating, what is the feeling you are getting from it? Does this place give you energy? Does it feel good? If it doesn't, reassure yourself that you are just sensing energy, and move to another spot.

Next, take your practice into your daily life. In what situations do you feel good and enlivened? With what people? Begin to tune in more often, and you will quickly learn where the energy drains are in your life. You may be surprised to find some people you spend time with often do not enhance your energy. You can now start to build more awareness, and down the road choose to separate yourself from people, places, and situations that deplete you. You are beginning to expand your life with knowledge of energy and practice sensing and working with it!

Clearing Your Energy

Clearing your energy field is a standard ritual that shamans use. When aiming to restore the field to its natural healed state, often the shaman finds debris or imprints from multiple encounters the person has had; thus, the field is not clear or clean and does not have impeccable boundaries. Each encounter during the day, each time someone thinks about you, each time you have an interaction with anything, your field is impacted to some degree. A residue of that interaction forms and often lingers. In modern-day shamanic terms, we refer to this as an imprint.

Often, a shaman wants to bring in higher-vibration, healed energy; however, they would not want to bring that energy into murky scaffolding, as adding fuel to an imprint will only aggravate its effect, so the first step is to clear the field.

Clearing is best done with a strong intention for the debris to float away. One way you could do clearing is to hold this intention, along with the image of your multicolored tapestry, then sweep your hands over your body. Clearing can also be done by visualizing pulling foreign energies from the field; you intuit what needs to be removed because it does not serve you.

These foreign energies can be transmuted by placing them in the transformative power of a fire. While visualizing, use your hands to move over your field, feeling and taking out the foreign energies and sending them to the flame of a candle. You can use a crystal or feather to wipe your field and then pass this object over the flame. If you do this, be sure you have cleared the crystal or feather. (You'll find instructions for doing this in chapter 12.)

Sending the unwanted energies away can be as "simple" as flicking the energy off your hands while intending that the energy goes to the fire and is combusted into an energy more useful to the Universe. Inherent in this practice is the assumption that an energy that might feel wrong or bad to you may be used by the Universe in a different way; therefore, we intend it to be transformed as opposed to destroyed.

In chapter 12, you will find exercises for clearing that are a bit more involved or focused on healing an imprint related to a specific health challenge. For now, practice these simpler versions. Clearing may be done many times, as our fields get congested with imprints from everyday life.

Shamanic Journeying to Achieve Awareness

I teach clients to access their deepest truth through journeying, also known as visualization or imagining. Shamanic journeying is closely related to hypnosis in that it involves a light trance that allows you to bypass the conscious mind and access the subconscious through experiencing a visualization. You move your awareness out of the literal world into the realm of possibilities. Self-hypnosis is easy and potent. When I trained as a hypnotherapist, I learned to record the scripts I had written and play them back to assist with my inner shifts.

Other valuable techniques for gaining insight and answers to questions are muscle testing and using a pendulum.

Muscle testing involves the assumption that if something approaches your energy field that is not good for the field, your muscles will be demonstrably weaker. Briefly, it involves stretching your arm out and holding the relevant item, such as sugar, sweetener, salt, and so forth, while the tester pushes down on the outstretched arm to test resistance: The greater the resistance, the better the substance is for the individual; the lower the resistance, the worse it is for them. In my experience, until you have good inner insight and body awareness, muscle testing is difficult to do by yourself.

On the other hand, using a pendulum can be done without anyone else's help. It involves holding a pendulum a few inches above a table, asking a yes or no question, and watching to see in which direction the pendulum moves. The direction of the movements—clockwise versus back and forth versus counterclockwise—are predetermined to mean accurate, maybe, or inaccurate.

I have found that if you are new to sensing energy, getting out of your thinking mind and surrendering to the answers that come to you while using a pendulum can be difficult. My own first attempts at using a pendulum were fraught with difficulties. First, I kept my eyes open, so it was hard to leave my thinking mind behind and go into a deeper space. Second, I did not always keep my arm relaxed, so I added to the energy of a direction when the pendulum started to move.

When I was first starting to learn to divine the truth of my situations, I lacked confidence and kept escaping back to my thinking mind. Before shamanic training, I spent my days in the scientific, academic world, and was very unsure about my intuition and its value. Even when I was able to relax and get information from using the pendulum, I kept negating those answers because it did not come with a scientific, provable evidence to back up what it was telling me. As a result, I decided to teach only through journeys and visualizations.

When someone journeys and gains information, any messages learned come from within. Much as they may try to discount the information, it is hard to dismiss that which is generated from within, so when they move to the steps that involve holding an intention, the actions come from within their thoughts. Our subconscious holds immense knowledge, and accessing it through journeying is very powerful, so it is good to get practice with shifting ways of seeing.

Let's start working with your imagination and embark on a visualization or journey. To record it for playback, you will need a small voice-activated recording device or software on your smartphone or computer. For example, if you use the program Zoom, you can save the file as an audio file only and label it as such.

Keep the script you have written next to you. Write one based on the instructions for journeys you find in this book, or use your imagination to create an original one. I suggest you include the following as key components of the script:

◊ An invocation to Spirit and any allies you have in order to open and enter sacred space. (This could be a prayer to God.)

◊ Instructions to relax, perhaps by focusing on the breath.

◊ Repetitive wording that can help you go deeper, deeper, deeper into relaxation.

◊ Directions to travel in your mind to a special place (such as a meadow, along a shoreline, on the peak of a mountain, or even the deepest space of your heart—use any setting that inspires you).

◊ Instructions to go deeper into that setting and make yourself comfortable there.

◊ A request for your Higher Self and a higher being or allies from the spirit realm to be present and answer questions for you. (You will meet and learn about these types of allies in the next chapter.)

◊ A meeting with a guide from whom you ask permission to do the work today or with whom you negotiate in order to learn what you need to do to gain permission. (This can help dissolve any hidden resistance to gaining insights that conflict with what you want to hear, setting you up to be open to suggestions to break out of your comfort zone of what you believe and how you act in your everyday life.)

◊ Any spaces within this special place you intend to interact with. (For example, you might journey with the intention of being presented with doors behind which lie answers you are seeking.)

◊ A question or questions to ask in this sacred space.

◊ A long pause, during which, in your mind's eye, you can see, feel, or know the answer, however it appears to you, and you might even want to leave time for continuing the dialogue if it feels right to do so (more on this momentarily).

◊ Instructions for offering gratitude to your spirit helpers before leaving.

◊ Instructions to mentally return to the present time and space, knowing that you may repeat the journey to gain further insights.

It is better to save any note taking until you are out of the visualization as you don't want to bring yourself into your literal mind, breaking the light hypnotic state. When you are finished asking for clarification, offer gratitude and move yourself (in your thoughts) back to the present time and space. Now sit and make notes on any insights you had, the information you received, the answers you got. Take notes while things are fresh in your mind; often something is lost if you move directly into your day's tasks and duties.

About the dialogue you will have (with your Wise One, Higher Self, or higher energy being) during the journey: When you have been given answers to the questions you had prepared to ask, you can take the discussion deeper by querying further. You can ask for clarification, requesting to be shown an image that will help you better understand the answer you were given. You can also ask about how you should proceed within the visualization or what you should do in your everyday life.

Consider asking for guidance with questions such as:

◊ What do I need to know about this health challenge?

◊ Is there something I need to change in my diet, and if so, what?

◊ What needs to shift in my lifestyle?

◊ Am I getting enough quality sleep, and if not, how do I shift this?

◊ Have I favored one part of my body over another, and if so, can you give me more information on that?

◊ What do I need to do to get back into physical balance?

◊ Is my body's movement sufficient, and if not, in what way do I change?

And:

◊ What do I need to know about the time I spend in joy and pleasure?

◊ What do I need to know about negative thoughts that need to change?

◊ What do I need to know about my burdens, duties, chores?

◊ Am I weighed down, and if so, what should I shift?

As well as:

◊ Are my relationships supportive and nourishing?

◊ If not, from whom do I need to separate or with whom do I need to change the dynamic between us?

And even:

◊ How should I improve my spiritual focus?

◊ Am I in a cage, and if so, what beliefs are trapping me?

Keep in mind that sometimes when you pose these questions, information will present itself in imagery and symbols. Sometimes you will have a knowing, rather than seeing something specific. Some people "hear" answers. However the insights come to you is perfectly fine.

○

Exercise

A Sample Shamanic Journey and Dialogue to Gain Awareness & Increase Intuition

Here is a simple script for a shamanic journey that will help you become aware by gaining insights. In future journeys, you can ask more pointed and deeper questions—or you can ask them during this journey and consider asking even more questions during another journey after you have taken notes on the answers you received initially and thought about them.

You might find that you have more questions. For example, in your first journey, you might ask what is out of balance and in what arena will your healing arise from. In future journeys, you might ask if the medication your physician prescribes will be enough to shift your health issue or whether something else should be integrated into your treatment (for example, acupuncture or adding more mushrooms to your diet, both of which can confer better immunity).

Feel free to change any of the sections to better suit you. If you record the text, use a relaxed voice that will assist you in going deeper into a state of awareness of what is unseen. Be sure to record some pauses so that when you are journeying you have enough time to process the images and symbols you see and messages you are given.

*[Start the recording and then
begin speaking the words written here.]*

- Begin by getting comfortable sitting or lying down. Take some nice deep, relaxing breaths in through your nose, out through your mouth. With each breath, feel yourself getting more and more relaxed . . . more and more relaxed.

[Pause]

- Move your awareness to the breath. Feel the breath enter and exit your body. With each breath, you are more and more relaxed.

[Pause]

- Let go of all the thoughts swirling through your mind. This is a time for entering deep relaxation, light trance, and accessing your subconscious. Allow the breath to carry you deeper and deeper.

[Pause]

- Allow all the tension to leave your body as you enter a space for gaining wisdom about _____ [state your health issue here].

[Pause]

- As you start this important journey to gain basic insight about _____ [state your health issue], declare this time and space that you are in to be sacred.

[Pause]

- Let's begin by calling to the winds of the South to come and bring light; calling to the winds of the West to come and bring courage; calling to the winds of the North to bring wisdom; calling to the winds of the East to bring a new view; calling to Mother Earth to support your endeavors; calling to Father Sky to light your way; calling on your Higher Self, your spirit guides, any guardian energies, any power animals you wish to be present.

[Pause]

- Now, travel in your mind's eye to a place that brings you peace, a place in which you are comfortable. Look around you, and take in all of the details of this special place.

[Pause]

- If you wish, you may make this your sacred space, and you may return at any time. Sit down and make yourself comfortable. As you get comfortable, maintain your relaxed state. Know that you are entering a space that is filled with wisdom, filled with insight, filled with information you can use for your personal growth.

  Ask that a Wise One comes forward. Perhaps this is your Higher Self, or an energy body or beam of light, or a guardian angel or spirit guide. Take in the details of this Wise One.

[Pause]

- Invite this Being/ Energy to sit down across from you. Offer your appreciation for its presence.

  Ask this Wise One to share with you something important for you to know about your health challenge. What do you need to know at this time? If the answer is not clear, ask for more details.

[Pause]

- At this time, what do you need to change in your life?

[Pause]

- Ask the Wise One for details of changes needed in the literal (physical) realm, the emotional realm, and the spiritual realm.

[Pause]

- If no answers come easily, take a deep breath. Are you relaxed enough? If not, take some nice, deep, relaxing breaths and let go of your thinking mind. Take yourself deeper and deeper.

[Pause]

- Now, ask again if there are changes needed in your physical, emotional, or spiritual realms.

[Pause]

- If no answers come forward, gather your courage. Ask the Wise One, "Am I ready to make changes?"

[Pause]

- If you are told that you are not ready, ask what you need to do to get ready to make changes.

[Pause]

- If you need more clarification, ask for more details.

[Pause]

- When information has stopped coming to you, ask if there is more to learn on this day. If you are told that this information is all for now, stop questioning and offer gratitude to the Wise One for coming forth today. Explain that you would like to come back another time to get more information.

[Pause]

- Before you leave, ask the Wise One for one more piece of assistance. Ask if it can speak more to you in your day-to-day life, and if so, could it be sure to use language or symbols you can understand. Ask that the messages you are sent be those that are clearly interpreted and heard by you.

[Pause]

- Bow in gratitude to the Wise One, and bring yourself back from your sacred place to the current time and place.

[Pause]

- Close sacred space by thanking and releasing the energies of the Four Directions, Mother Earth, and Father Sky. Winds of the South, thank you for being here. Winds of the West, thank you for bringing courage. Winds of the North, thank you for your wisdom. Winds of the East, thank you for bringing a new perspective. Mother Earth, thank you for supporting me. Father Sky, thank you for shining the light on my days.

- Come back to the current time and place and open your eyes. While you are still in a meditative state, begin journaling or writing down important messages you received.

[Stop recording]

Did you take the journey? Good job! You have now learned how to sense energy, how to restore your energy body, and how to begin to connect with energy fields in your day-to-day life. You have learned how to write, record, and take a meditative journey to your inner world, where vast amounts of information exist. You have gleaned details of the first layers of your health challenge and have now seen where this issue exists in the physical, the emotional, and the spiritual. And you have practiced moving out of your intellectual, rational head space into the intuitive, sensing world.

Commit to doing the exercises in this chapter so that you can truly become more aware of what information and insights are available to you and learn to work with your energy body. Let's move now to the next step in which you will *Allow* outside assistance in healing and *Amplify* your potential for a healed outcome.

Allow

After you have entered a deeper awareness of aspects of your health challenge and done some intuitive exploring through journeying and working with your luminous energy field, the next step is to get some power behind your desire to shift.

I know firsthand the helpless feeling of being acutely and vividly aware of something that is not working as it should and not believing you are capable of changing it. When we are locked inside our minds, with our human perspective, which is flawed and limited, many things seem beyond our control, beyond our potential to shift. Being in that position is incredibly anxiety producing.

I grew up in a household of intensity, anger, mental illness, and alcoholism. Additionally, my family was living overseas in non-English speaking countries and moving households every 18 months to two years, which was stressful for me. Every two years, I had to reorient to a new school, try to make new friends, and try to fit in as a blonde, white-skinned minority. When I now reflect on how my default traits came to be hypervigilant and guarded, I find myself asking,

"Is it any wonder?"

When I was younger, I turned to animals, finding them easy to meet and get along with. I also turned to my intellect, striving to get good grades, master the material, and be the teacher's pet. As I got older, I began to see the one-sidedness of my traits—my anxiety, my worries. Despite my academic achievements, my anxiety never left.

Every now and then, without my bidding, something would happen to me that could be categorized as "woo-woo." At these times, I felt pushed to learn about the unseen world of psychic phenomena, lucid dreams, intuition, and the magic kingdom. How did my mom know exactly what present I had bought her for Christmas and how it was wrapped, even though I had never talked about the gift and had hidden it well? How did I fly in my dreams to another geographic location, travel down to see the details on the land, and later have a friend confirm the details, because in real life, she had been in that very location at the time I was asleep?

How did I know to awaken one May night at 10:30 p.m. (my bedtime is 8:30!) to look out over the front yard, where I saw a large group of small lights shooting back and forth from out of the woods, moving like a cloud across the front yard and garden at an unbelievable speed? And why, despite being a little fearful, did I wake up the next few nights, look out into the pitch black, and ask that the lights return—and after some five minutes of heartfelt asking, they did? How did that happen again and again for several nights in a row, for several Mays in a row?

All these unusual experiences happened because I allowed myself to tap into what is hidden from ordinary consciousness and amplify my perspective and relationship to the unseen. I released any fear about the unknown and trusted that the Universe would protect me.

When I was first studying shamanism, I traveled to Sedona, Arizona, with a group of like-minded women for a spiritual retreat. One day, we took a planned hike up the red rocks with our guide, Jaap van Etten, Ph.D., who is a deep metaphysician. Jaap took us to certain places that he, as a result of insights and experiences he has had while meditating there, has determined to be vortexes on energy lines, or ley lines, on Earth.

Jaap sat our group down on a mesa top in the April sun and led us in a meditation designed to connect us with energetic forces of creation deep inside the earth that he intuits as dragons. Jaap has built relationships with these beings, so he specifically asked one to come forth to meet the group.[19] Many times, dragons are portrayed as frightening, but Jaap introduced them as deep energies of the earth. Because I was sitting in a spiritual circle amid the beauty of the red rocks of Sedona and am very connected to the earth, I think that is why I felt no fear.

After the meditation, we all shared our experiences. I said that I had felt a current of power coming from deep within the earth and visualized it as a large celadon-green female dragon. She was calm and non-aggressive, but I could sense that she had immense power and that she could be ferocious and lethal. My intellectual mind was recalling how in Chinese mythology the dragon is a revered being, representing good fortune and having authority over forces of nature, such as typhoons.

My left brain went on to explain this phenomenon of meeting dragons: As humans, we need to give structure and explanation to forces of nature and currents of geologic power, and we are good at anthropomorphizing everything. Our group had been told that we were to meet a dragon, so this is likely why I then visualized this power in this form. It all made sense, but I could not shake how I felt as that current of energy poured over and into me. I genuinely felt that it was not just a geologic force but a dragon.

Afterward, I began to connect daily to that feeling I'd had, keeping the name "dragon" as I consciously asked that this energy join me in my thoughts and my endeavors.

A week or so later, back at home, I was doing a shamanic energy session with my sister, and without words, I asked the dragon to come help shift my sister's condition toward the desired outcome. I visualized the celadon-green female dragon assisting, but also saw two smaller, younger dragons that were cobalt-blue and greenish-blue.

When the session was over, my sister reported feeling shifts that were very powerful.

I said, "I bet they were—I asked the dragon to help." (I had told her about my experience with Jaap van Etten.)

My sister replied: "Yes, it was there—a large pale-green dragon—but there also were two other smaller dragons."

You can imagine my thrill of having such confirmation of the presence of unseen forces!

The more I opened to accept the intangible and to recognize that there are immense powers in the unseen world, the more my anxiety dissipated. I sought metaphysical and mystical studies that offered explanation of the world outside myself. What I learned has shown me that humans can align with and build alliances with the forces of Nature and the Universe. My experiences with the inhabitants of Earth (animal, plants, and elements) have shown me an intelligent interconnectedness.

As I aligned spiritually, I began to have a new faith—that I am not alone and have allies that can amplify the work I do here on Earth in unseen realms.

Meeting Helpers

After gaining an increasing amount of insight into the matter, the next step in shifting your health challenge is to gather the power to make a shift. You do that at step 2 on the Wheels of Inner Tasks and Actions: You *Allow* and *Amplify*.

This is the point on your spiral journey for you to ally with forces and beings that will serve as your helpers. If your human potential could give you all the power you need to make the shift in your health issue, it likely would have happened by now. At this point, go big, don't hold back in reaching out. Allow the amplification efforts of the "big guns"—Spirit in different forms.

If you grew up in a monotheistic religion, bear with me as I introduce you to another way of thinking about how Spirit operates. It appears that every indigenous culture has its creatures of magical and mystical powers, including angels. Throughout the ages, stories of these unseen beings abound. Icelanders describe hidden folk, akin to elves. Celtic culture describes many forms of fairies—leprechauns, banshees, gnomes—and each category has different characteristics. African cultures describe many deities, some more powerful than others. These beings represent different energetic qualities, which you can experience as you connect with them in meditation. A dragon usually exhibits a powerful, deep energetic current, while a garden *deva* may have a lighter quality.

The naming and categorizing of unseen magical creatures has been written off as a human need to gain some emotional control over and explanation of unexpected and sometimes frightening events; however, in shamanic work, practitioners ally themselves with Nature spirits, power animals, and other energies and intelligences, all of which you might think of as Spirit in some form.

How can connecting with unseen beings benefit us in our healing? The Universe is filled with complex energetics. If we can bring different energies into our luminous energy field, and if we can resonate with them, harmonizing with their vibration, we have the potential to shift and improve the energetics of our current field.

When we connect with the Universal Field, we have access to vast, expansive, dynamic energies outside ourselves. When we access the transcendental realms, we are stepping out of human limitations and into a place of infinite possibility perfect for shifting a health challenge. We enter this place through the right brain, the feeling and intuitive side that is too often ignored by Western medicine.

Imagine your knee is stiff and inflexible from arthritis. If you could flood your field with a flexible, sinewy energy, perhaps visualized as a water dragon or water nymph, you would be resonating with that type of energy and subsequently changing your energetics to be more fluid.

If your knee is badly inflamed, connecting with an energy or being that exemplifies peace would likely be beneficial as well.

When you were feeling the colors in your luminous field while doing the Colors exercise in the previous chapter, you may have also felt that they had different qualities of energies. In fact, color does have a wavelength and hence, a frequency. Each of the helpers described below has its own unique energetic signature, if you will. When you connect with each of them, you will likely sense the difference in energy—deep and grounding (meaning solid and feeling earth connected) or perhaps light and ethereal (meaning a wispy sense, more floating than earth connected). The more you connect, the easier it will be for you to tell the differences in the energy of various helpers:

◊ Your Higher Self

◊ Your ancestors

◊ Power animals

◊ Elemental and nature spirits

◊ Dragons

◊ Ascended masters

◊ Angels, Mother Mary, Master Jesus

As you practice allowing yourself to encounter and interact with these allies, I am sure you will come to appreciate and even love those energetic differences. After I describe some common helpers, I will share practices that can make it easier for you to connect with them.

As you work at allowing and amplifying, it's important to know that there are low-quality energies in the world, sometimes described as "dark forces." When you enter a meditative space, you might connect with energies that are powerful but do not engender feelings that are essential for healing. In my thinking, healing happens in an energetic field that is one of compassion, tolerance, unity, love, and so forth. If you do not *feel* good when encountering a particular energy, do not connect. You are the ultimate guardian of your energy field.

Your Higher Self

Earlier, I introduced you to your Higher Self, which is your inner core: the eternal, conscious, and intelligent you. It is the form of your being that is in connection with the Divine, with Source, with All That Is. In most cases, your Higher Self is the Wise One you access when you are doing self-hypnosis and undertaking journeys. Your Higher Self can offer you insights that are hidden from your conscious mind.

Your Ancestors

Many people believe that we exist after death, in the afterlife. Further, many people believe that our ancestors in the afterlife can still influence our lives. Regardless of whether you believe in the afterlife, through meditation, you can connect with the energies that your ancestors hold. Doing this can be especially impactful when you are dealing with an illness that has a heritable component.

Power Animals

Shamans of many cultures work closely with power animals, also known as spirit animals. As you learned earlier, shamanism is animistic: Shamans believe that all animals, creatures, places—and in fact, all things that are part of the natural world—are interconnected. In shamanic traditions, each animal has specific characteristics attributed to it.

For example, shamans might say a dolphin power animal has intelligent and playful energy, while a wolf exemplifies social connections, loyalty, and guardianship, and a jaguar is courageous and fierce and can track its path in the dark using other senses.

You might want to learn more about power animals by reading Ted Andrews' *Animal Speak: The Spiritual & Magical Powers of Creatures Great and Small*. It's an excellent compilation of the qualities associated with animals, based on what Andrews and others have intuited about their nature and how they can help us. Andrews writes:

The early priest/ess–magicians would adopt the guise of animals—wearing skins and masks—to symbolize a reawakening and endowing of oneself with specific energies . . . To them, every species and every aspect of the environment had the power to remind them of what they could manifest within their own life. It was an aid to bridge the natural worlds to the supernatural, awakening the realities of both within the environs of their own lives.[20]

The benefit of connecting with a power animal is that you can work with that particular animal's qualities. You can start by reading about it, keeping pictures of it around you, and sensing what it would be like to embody its characteristics. In journeys to retrieve a power animal, the animal that appears to you is one that offers you energies you need for your life or for tasks ahead or energies you may not express well within yourself. Author and spiritual teacher Alberto Villoldo teaches that allying with a power animal is about who you are becoming, not who you would like to be. Working with a power animal can help you bring about change because it can offer its qualities to you.

Elementals and Nature Spirits

As far back as the 16th century, and in today's New Age mysticism, elemental energies have been associated with each of the four elements: Earth, Air, Fire, and Water (with Metal sometimes considered an element, too).

I have a more generalized interpretation of these natural energies. I connect with different energies associated with the land I live on—energies of the vegetable garden, energies of the woods, energies of the stream, energies of the flowers. Each of these feels different to me when I take myself out of ordinary awareness and tap into them. And when I do connect, I feel part of a bigger world; that is, the world of the trees or the brook or the flowers.

Many indigenous tribes connect deeply with the land itself—with the soil and with the energy lines (ley lines) along the earth's surface. For example, Mayan pyramids were built along unmarked roads extending from them—roads that could only be seen energetically. Australian Aboriginals walk "song lines;" that is, they follow unseen tracks through the desert that they remember because of ancient, sacred songs sung to them about the geography and mystical importance of each path.

So, for me, elementals are more than the actual elements of Earth, Air, Fire, and Water; they have different energies, any of which we can work with to attain better health and well-being.

Dragons

As I have written above, the dragons I work with are powerful energies and intimately connected with the forces of the earth and creativity. Dragons of different realms exist within the elements of Fire, Water, Earth, and Air, and in the celestial not just earth realms.

Diana Cooper, a gifted intuitive and mystic, has written a book on the work she has done with dragons and shares practical knowledge about dragons. She has intuited multiple aspects of dragons—earth energy, celestial energy, energies of the different elements (Water, Fire, Earth, and Air). "Dragons are extremely sage, courageous, open-hearted beings who have been serving our planet from its inception . . . Dragons are part of our ancient history, so knowing them is encoded into our memory banks."[21]

I am partial to those dragon energies that arise from the earth. I feel them as a deep rumbling energy. I sense them flowing up from beneath me, and I am usually in Nature when I connect with them. This contrasts with the times I have connected with celestial dragons, which seem to me to be a lighter, wispier energy. They are contacted from the space above me, and I experience a lifting sense, rather than a grounding sense.

Ascended Masters

Some people who have connected with ascended masters feel they are beings that have previously been in human form but have achieved spiritual enlightenment through overcoming karma. Karma is defined as "The sum of a person's actions in this and previous states of existence, viewed as deciding their fate in future existences."[22] It is not necessary to believe in the spiritual ideas behind the description of the ascended masters. In essence, if a being (or energy) is of a high vibrational quality, holding properties of peace/love/joy/serenity, then I find it valuable to connect with it and don't need to decide whether it is an ascended master or some other type of helper.

Angels, Mother Mary, Master Jesus

The beings in this category have their origin in Christianity, but you do not have to be Christian to benefit from their vibrational field. The qualities of these spiritual beings are those of love and devotion.

Both Mother Mary and Master Jesus are believed to have achieved very high vibrational fields and enlightened spirituality, making for powerful allies for healing. Angels are said to have never taken human form, which supports the idea that they are of higher vibration than spirit guides, which are usually energies that had previously taken human form. (Humans operate in the material world, and thus their fields interact and resonate with multiple frequencies.)

Working as a physician in COVID-19 times has been particularly trying. Many patients are filled with anxiety, anger, and helplessness. It has been a struggle for me to stay tolerant in many situations, especially if I hold certain beliefs about science and COVID and my patients do not.

As I found myself getting more and more irritable and testy, I began to work with the energy of Mother Mary. To me, Mary represents the ultimate of love and compassion. I used roses as a symbol of those energies. So, for at least a few weeks, multiple times a day, when confronted with something that raised my ire, I consciously thought about roses and asked for Mary to help me drop my irritability. When a situation was unbearable, I asked for an image of a blanket of roses to drop over me and the situation and sensed that blanket landing over me like a comforting quilt. I bought rosewater spray to spritz myself with the scent of roses to help me energetically experience the blanket of roses soothing me. My aggravation eased, my mood improved, and my tolerance grew. Thank you to the energy of Mary!

Practices to Connect with Helpers

Let's take some time to connect with earth-centered energies, power animals, and energies from the more ethereal, celestial realms. These practices can be adapted for you to tap into any being you choose.

Note: There are many energies to connect with in the Universal Field, so there may come a time when you encounter a force you are not comfortable with. Remember: If the energy does not feel good, or if you feel that you are being intruded upon, firmly state that your energy field is your own and that you are sovereign, and command the entity to leave you alone. Your field is completely under your control. Knowing and believing this will protect you—just as knowing and believing is the best way to achieve healing.

Exercise

Connect with a Power Animal

This practice is an adaptation of a shamanic journey adapted from class teachings of the Four Winds Society. You will open and close space, and at the end offer gratitude. You will travel to the Underworld, where you will meet a power animal. In the shamanic tradition of the Andes, as well as in other spiritual traditions, the Underworld is not evil; rather, it is the place of your subconscious, where things may be hidden from your awareness. In traveling to the Underworld, you can learn much information that may have previously been unknown.

In Peruvian cosmology, the caretaker of the Underworld is Huascar (pronounced Waa-Skar). You might think of him as a protector and guide for this journey. The Tree of Life (World Tree) is a fundamental archetype concept in many shamanic cultures—having roots in Earth with branches reaching to Sky (connecting Heaven to Earth). You will be engaging both Huascar and the Tree.

Note that in the description of the Underworld journey, I include statements within the script for the visualization that suggest positive experiences. For example, I say, "You know you will find something important here" or "You know that valuable information is ahead." As the visualization is engaging your subconscious, it is important to set the tone and steer the experience so that the journey will allow you to retrieve valuable information. When you write your own scripts for journeys, be sure to include positive suggestive statements.

[Start recording]

- Make yourself comfortable by sitting comfortably or lying down. Close your eyes. Bring yourself into a relaxed state by following your breath. Breathe in through your nose, out through your mouth. Allow each breath to take you deeper and deeper. More and more relaxed.

[Pause]

- Allow your awareness to travel to your heart space. Remain relaxed, with comfortable breaths.

[Pause]

144

- Now move your awareness out of your body, and find yourself walking in a luscious meadow on a beautiful, sunny day. As you walk, you know that you are heading toward something important. You know that you are about to gain some knowledge or understanding that will be very helpful for you.

- Ahead of you in the middle of the meadow is a large, beautiful tree. You sense its wisdom and power. As you get closer to this tree, you see the solid, large trunk and parts of the larger roots extending out of the ground. The tree's branches extend high into the clouds. You notice a hole in the base of the tree. You feel drawn to the wisdom and power here. Curious, you dive into the hole and begin to travel down through the bedrock, through the layers of soil and rock, following the tree roots.

[Pause]

- You travel deeper and deeper into the earth, past the roots, and passing some veins of quartz and other gemstones. And now, you find you have arrived at the side of an underground stream.

[Pause]

- You are drawn to the stream, knowing that it is leading you to important knowledge. You comfortably step into it and lie down to float and be carried along in its currents. The stream moves you downstream. As you float with the water washing around you, you sense that barriers to your understanding are being released. Down and down you go, farther downstream, until the current slows and you arrive at a sandy bank.

[Pause]

- You call to Huascar, the guardian of this place, to ask permission to visit, knowing he is a protective ally to journeyers.

[Pause]

- Huascar appears from the trees along the stream. Notice his appearance. Introduce yourself, and ask if now is a good time to visit.

- If Huascar says no, ask if there is anything you need to say or do to make this a good time to visit. If he still says no, that today is not a good day, trust his judgment. Remember, he wants to keep you safe and see that you have a positive, powerful experience in the Underworld. Don't fret if Huascar denies you permission to continue going into the Underworld. Some days are not energetically good for journeys. This does not mean that you cannot try again another day.If you don't have Huascar's permission, even after negotiating with him, it's best to return to the stream.

[Pause]

- Once you are at the stream again, travel back up the bedrock, back up the roots of the tree, and come out of the base of the tree. Then walk back into this current time and place.

- If you are still in the Underworld, and Huascar has granted you access to travel farther, tell him that you have come to meet a power animal with whom you want to establish an important relationship. Ask Huascar to assist you in meeting this animal.

[Pause]

- You look up from the bank of the stream into the grove of trees along the bank. Out of the trees comes a power animal.

[Pause]

- Observe which animal appears. If more than one appears, notice which animal is coming forward the closest to you, indicating that it wants to engage with you. If an insect appears, even a butterfly, thank it for its presence, and simply observe it.

- When one animal makes its presence known and steps forward to you, see it or feel it or sense it—however you connect with it.

[Pause]

- What energies do you feel emanate from this animal?

[Pause]

- With Huascar overseeing the conversation, ask this animal what message it brings for you.

[Pause]

- What capacities does this animal have that are important for you now?

[Pause]

- What can this animal teach you?

  [Pause]

- Ask more questions, including questions for clarification. Have a dialogue to learn more about the energies this animal brings forward.

- Next, dialogue with the animal to learn how it will share its wisdom with you and how it can offer you a new way of being.

  [Pause]

- Find out how it will get your attention in your day-to-day life for you to hear the wisdom it offers. Perhaps you establish that the animal will appear as an image in your awareness, at which point you know to slow down and hear what it has to say. Perhaps you establish a code word that it will use to make you stop and listen. And, of course, ask what it would want from you in return.

  [Pause]

- Next, ask the animal if it will come back with you to your literal world and assist you in healing and living a better life.

  [Pause]

- If the animal says no or hesitates, ask if there is something you need to do or change to have this animal join you.

  [Pause]

- Once you have negotiated passage out of the Underworld for the animal, have it move close to you, then step back into the stream. Notice that it accompanies you. You and the animal then travel upstream and exit into the bedrock. Travel up through the strata of rock and gemstone, to the roots of the tree, and up to exit out of the base of the tree. Walk back out of the meadow, the animal at your side, back to the current time and place.

  [Stop recording]

Back in the literal world, you need to keep this relationship with the power animal alive. Nothing sends a power animal packing (leaving you) more quickly than being undervalued, not listened to, or ignored. Put up pictures of the animal around your meditation room or house. Take quiet time to feel and talk to the animal daily. And, of course, when talking, make sure you balance asking for its help with offering gratitude and asking what you may do in return. The energies a power animal can bring you are potent and life changing; honor and respect the relationship you create.

As part of the Healing the Light Body curriculum at the Four Winds Society, we were taught to develop relationships with the four main archetypes of Peruvian cosmology: Serpent, Jaguar, Hummingbird, and Eagle (or Condor). We worked with each archetype for some weeks, deepening our connection.

I was driving home from one of our workshops, on a highway that was relatively free of traffic, after doing a workshop focused on the archetype of Eagle. For me, living in the Eastern United States, I find that Hawk serves as the representative of Eagle or Condor, and I had begun to connect with Hawk and come to love its power of big sight, of soaring above the mundane, of clear, discerning vision. I was driving on a sunny day, and there was no one else on the road around me.

Bam! Something hit my windshield, coming in diagonally from high on the left, moving rapidly downward to the right. I saw feathers tumble across the windshield, and I braked with panic and anxiety. I knew that a hawk had hit my car, and I was devastated that I had killed a member of my power animal team. I pulled over to the side and backed up a little to where I had seen the hawk tumble to the shoulder of the road.

There was no hawk anywhere. I saw feathers and a little blood on the windshield, but despite searching the shoulder and grass border, I could not find a hawk.

Shaken, I got back into the car and drove on. Within a mile I came upon a multicar accident that obviously had just occurred. Two cars were totaled. Astonished, I knew that had I been on this stretch of road 5–10 minutes earlier, I would have been involved in this deadly crash. Remembering my burgeoning relationship, I felt an upwelling of deep gratitude for Hawk. Had Hawk not hit my car, I would not have been delayed and may have been badly injured or even dead. I offered my profound apologies for any injury to Hawk and renewed my commitment to being allies.

Through the years since, many times when I am driving, accompanied by my girlfriend, in mystical conversation, Hawk will appear on a phone line we pass or fly overhead. I then am lifted to the Hawk energy of big sight, of expansive soaring, of keen discerning vision, and I remember its protectiveness toward me when it could see what I could not.

○

Exercise
Connect to a Celestial Being

On this journey, you will travel to and connect with a being in the celestial realm. The realm you will connect with is that of angels and ascended masters, of enlightened ones that can serve as a divine guide for you.

An enlightened being is one that exhibits the purest of qualities (integrity, compassion, love, peace, benevolence, truth, and so on) and that is close in its nature to the Divine (Source). This means that a being or energy from this realm has knowledge of life and the power of manifesting: It can bring something tangible into your life as a result of your thoughts and belief. The value of connecting with a being such as this is to bring your field into resonance with these illuminated qualities.

[Start recording]

- Make yourself comfortable by sitting comfortably or lying down. Close your eyes. Bring yourself into a relaxed state by following your breath. Breathe in through your nose, out through your mouth. Allow each breath to take you deeper and deeper. Become more and more relaxed.

- Let yourself focus your awareness on the insides of your eyelids. Next, bring your awareness down from your eyes, through your head, down behind your throat, down into your neck, and arrive in your chest.

[Pause]

- Staying relaxed, with comfortable breaths, move your awareness inside your chest to your heart. Sense or feel or know how to find the sacred space of your heart. Here is the center of streams of energy coming in and traveling out of your field. Find yourself traveling into the heart, to the sacred space of your heart.

[Pause]

- As you arrive here, you know that you are heading for something important. You know that deep wisdom and understanding are just ahead.

[Pause]

- Enter the room in the space of your heart. This is a sacred place where your soul connects with Spirit. Look around the room, and see its richness and beauty. Find a comfortable place to sit. Then, center yourself in this space of your essence.

[Pause]

- Next, visualize a golden cord of light leaving your heart and traveling down, through your body, out your feet, deep into the earth. Feel the energy of that cord, carrying your love and connection to the earth. Now feel the energy the earth sends you, coming up the golden cord to your heart.

[Pause]

- Know of your deep relationship with the earth.

- Now send the golden cord of light from your heart space to the heavens. Feel the energy traveling up from your heart to the enlightened realms. These are the realms of divine intelligence, of your galactic connections. Send your energy up the cord to the heavens, and feel the energies returning to you. As you sit with the golden cord running through you, know what the ancient shamans knew—that you are the center of a sacred trinity of human, Earth, and Sky. Know that your luminous field is constantly informed by shifts and energies of Earth and Sky.

[Pause]

- Bring your awareness back to the room in which you are sitting, in the sacred space of your heart. Ask that an energy or being of the highest order come forward to be present with you. This is an energy of higher potency than the Wise One, more powerful than any power animal. Feel the space around you as this energy comes in.

[Pause]

- Take in the details of what you see, feel, sense, or know. Sense the benevolent guidance of this energy. Feel yourself humbled in the presence of this greatness.

[Pause]

- Now, bring your health challenge to your awareness. Feel a representation of this challenge move onto your outstretched hands. Now, holding your health challenge, place it at the feet of this divine guide. Feel yourself surrender your health challenge to this omnipotent energy. Truly and completely release control of your issue. Take stock of the emotions and thoughts that wash over you as you turn your issue over to something far bigger than yourself.

[Pause]

- Now start a conversation with this guide. Ask for assistance in navigating a shift from a lack to wholeness, from damaged to complete and repaired. Ask to be able to hear guidance in your day-to-day life, to make correct decisions and wise choices.

[Pause]

- Sense a golden light of powerful healing energy coming from this guide. Allow this light to fill the sacred space of your heart. Feel the healing light surround you and enter your field—top to bottom, front to back, outside to inside. Sit for a few moments in this golden light, knowing you are being restored, rejuvenated, replenished.

[Pause]

- Know that you can return here anytime to connect with this divine guide.

- Now, offer your gratitude to this energy for being present. Bow in appreciation to the sacred space of your heart. With your awareness, make your way out of the heart, back up from the chest, back to the view from behind your eyes. Bring yourself back to the current time and place, and open your eyes.

[Stop recording]

You might be thinking: *Why are you teaching me to master my field, when at the same time you have just told me to surrender? What gives? Am I taking charge or am I surrendering?*

Yes, it does seem confusing. The answer is both. You are being taught to master your thoughts and your inner awareness—things that exist in the human realm. These are within your limited human purview.

Increased awareness and mastery make these processes less limited, but you are still operating within the human capacity. When you surrender, allowing helpers to amplify your power, you are surrendering to the vast potential of the Universe, to an intelligence greater than yourself. You are calling in and connecting with expanded wisdom and power. In other words, you are being asked to become a master of your human form—its thoughts and personal field—but also asking for help in allying with the magnitude and pulse of life force itself.

You are gaining it all—expanded human resonating with the Divine. This expanded capacity, as a result of joining with forces greater than yourself and aligning yourself with elevated thoughts of self-compassion, peace, and truth, brings you power on your journey to shift a health challenge.

In closing this chapter, I will share a personal story of surrender. All my life I have valued control. With the dysfunction I grew up in, my way of coping was to be very tightly wound, to ensure I was safe within my ability to command. When I was first learning shamanic energy practices, I worked hard at extending my connections outside myself, to allow help from other sources. Truthfully, I found it easier to accept help from a power animal, as I resonated with animals.

In one session with a client whose issue was particularly challenging, I found myself at a loss for answers. I knew I needed *big* help. I then allowed (operative word: *Allow!*) my awareness to travel to the Sky realm and ask for assistance from something big. I admitted that I was at a loss, that I knew nothing, and I *surrendered* to the vast expanse outside of myself.

Then came the shocker! I felt a rush of energy pour in through my head and out my hands. When I looked at my hands, there was a shimmer and vibrating glow that extended an inch or more from each of my fingertips. As I watched, I realized I was no longer in charge.

The vibration moved across the client's body without me directing the process. I saw the glow push the pain and struggle out of the client's body. The entire shift took less than five minutes and then was over. My awareness returned to my human thoughts, and I completed the session.

The client was stunned by how good he felt, how for the first time in as long as he could remember, his pain was gone. His health challenge shifted, and he experienced wholeness. He has stayed shifted. Bottom line: The Big Guns are out there, and they are powerful! Use them!

You have now learned how to cultivate an ally and how to use its power to assist you. You have been reminded to hold respect for these energies and to remain in *ayni* (right relation) by offering gratitude. In the next chapter we will move to the next steps: *Act* and *Intention*.

11

Act with Intention

You are well on your way in the journey of shifting your health challenge! So far, I hope that your exploration of the concepts and practices I described in earlier chapters has been fun and exciting and that you have been able to sense the power these practices bring. The inner work you do is key to your spiritual expansion, and this spiritual expansion is a (if not the) potent driver of your physicality.

We move now into step 3 on our wheels of Inner Tasks and Inner Actions. This is the step where you clearly state your deepest desire for your health. It's where you sing it to the rooftops (metaphorically)—from the place of your soul's essence/Higher Self—that you intend to shift your health challenge for the better.

The key concepts here are to *Act* and with *Intention*. Briefly, taking action is almost always a good step, particularly as you get nowhere when sitting at the fork in the road, donkey-like, undecided, paralyzed by inaction. Now, I am not going to argue that simply *being* is not valuable and that quiet time is not essential to our sanity; however, I will argue that if you want to shift your health challenge, staying in the undecided without a plan takes you nowhere.

Up until this point in the book, you have been deepening into the quiet to gather more data about your health issue (*Aware*) and then aligning yourself with powerful forces (*Allow*), and, you have seen the power of your thoughts and energy field. So, now, we will focus those thoughts into an intention for improved health, well-being, and freedom from limitation.

What is *Intention?*

As I said earlier, I see *Intention* as an energy, a straight arrow of intense wishing, aiming at the target of your desired outcome. Anyone can shoot arrows of thought; the potency comes from choosing an arrow laden with energies specific and perfect for your goal and aiming it at the target you actually want.

How then do you make an intention perfect? The answer lies in how you *feel* when you visualize yourself at the arrow's end of that thought. Let me give you some examples.

In her book *The Amazing Power of Deliberate Intent,* Esther Hicks suggests using how you feel to determine if your stated intention is the right one for you. You can use negative feelings to steer you toward the intention you do want. In other words, when you imagine yourself experiencing the outcome of your intention, if that future experience you're imagining does not feel good and perfect to you, reconfigure the original intention.[23]

Let's say that you want your lower back to stop hurting. As you look ahead to how that wish might play out, you see that you may end up with a surgery that fuses your vertebrae, which alleviates the pain but worsens your flexibility, which, in turn, makes you feel frustrated and sad. Recognizing this, you would want to revise your intention to include reduction of pain and improvement in mobility.

Or let's say that you are overweight and have knee pain. Sometimes when you walk, you feel a stabbing pain on the outside of your knee, so you walk less. Your orthopedic doctor has told you that your weight is a contributor to the arthritis you have in your knee. Once again, as society has done so many times before, you are reminded about how bad you are for being overweight, and this leads to you being angry at yourself for being fat, so you intend to lose weight to help your knees. Every night before going to bed, you scold yourself for what you ate that day, vow to do better, and fall asleep hating yourself and mad at your body. You say, "I intend to stop being so fat so that my knees are better."

Your arrows of thought are laden with anger, self-loathing, and your soul and body are in conflict. Can you feel healing in this situation? Can you feel a path of uplift and expansion? Do you feel a powerful energy field arising from this situation? I think not.

Here is another illustration of why the above approach is not an effective one. Imagine yourself on the road ahead in your healing journey as you think the thoughts of how terrible you are for being fat, how mad you are at your knees and your fat body, and how you need to change, because you are a flawed, defective person.

As you look ahead on this path, do you see yourself standing in bright sunlight? Is your human figure glowing with connection between Spirit and your essence? Does that future You seem healed? I am going to bet that as you struggle to see yourself as changed, lifted out of your current pain and limitations, the imagery is hard to hold onto because you are spinning around with chaotic, self-despising energies. I also will bet that you cannot clearly see a healed You.

Instead, let's ask ourselves, *What is the real goal here?* For you, it might be to have less pain, to be more active, and to feel good about yourself as you walk through the world. What, then, is the feeling state you should embody as you send your arrows of thoughts forward?

Consider this feeling state: a sense of appreciation for your skeletal structure as it carries you in the world, an excitement about walking without pain and with flexibility, encouragement to listen to *all* of your body and to involve *all* of you in resolving this situation, and excitement about choosing foods that reduce inflammation, with the side benefit of helping weight fall away.

Now, your intention might be "I intend to listen to and honor all parts of my body" or "I intend to operate in internal harmony, with my body and Spirit working together" or "I intend to be pain-free, so I make choices that honor and support me." Perhaps a more specific intention could be "I intend to bring healing to my knees." Inherent in this last intention statement is the assumption that "healing" is the experience of feeling uplifted, of sunlight and expansion and wisdom, of your body working in its best form and in harmony.

Now, let's imagine your future self as energized, alive, powerful, limber, active, and happy to be alive. Wow! What a difference! Now, as you fall asleep each night, you flood your mind with thoughts of being in harmony within your body, of being a new revitalized You, of bringing forth all your personal power in concert with your spiritual allies to shift your pain and limited mobility. You can feel yourself moving forward into that new and improved state, and you feel good.

Feeling

As you have seen from the examples above, how you *feel* while holding certain thoughts is important to choosing how you focus your intention, remembering that creative qualities, such as peace, joy, love, bliss, forgiveness, acceptance, willingness, and courage, trump destructive qualities, such as anger, fear, despair, grief, blame, shame, and humiliation.

The feelings you hold in your awareness change the vibrational quality of your energy field. You can intuitively understand that your cellular machinery will work better under energetic conditions flooded with creative qualities. Remembering the Maximum Medicine Mind Matrix, in your awareness you want the expanded and revitalized energies of consciousness.

There is one tricky emotion or feeling that deserves at least a short discussion. That is the emotion of desire, or strong longing. Here is why this emotion is tricky and best to stay away from when generating your healing intentions. For the most part, when we are feeling strong desire, we are overcome with a longing that springs from the platform of what we don't have already. A platform of "don't have," or lack, is not a good platform from which to send out our healing intentions. The underpinnings are those of feeling loss, or lack, or feeling not good enough to have something. In other words, in most situations, when we are desiring something strongly, it is because we are deeply aware that we do not have that something. Underneath the desire is the ever-present awareness of something not right, something wrong, something not good enough; of energies that are not of the highest vibrational quality and that do not lead to expanded potential for healing. It is tricky to create intentions from a place of desire; I recommend you avoid this.

You might ask, "How can I avoid feeling desire, and therefore, lack, when I am so strongly wishing that my health challenge would resolve itself?" "How can I not desire to be free of these limitations?"

For most of us standing at life's major choice points and wishing to step onto a healing path, there is the strong desire to *not* be on the path we are on at that time; indeed, the desire to change is a very strong driver of new choices. So you might ask, "How can you tell me to not feel that?"

I know that you feel that strong desire, and I know that you have the drive to change. When seeing the "other side of the fence," you are acutely aware of the grass you are standing on this side of the fence.

I find the trick is to step beyond the desire that has pushed you to make changes. By "step beyond," I mean feeling your way into the space you want to occupy—a space that is expanded, vital, energized, whole, healed, and buzzing with life force. Feel yourself to be whole, healed, and alive.

You might not feel this way at all when you begin, so use the power and creativity of your thoughts. Imagine and visualize—paint a picture of who you see yourself as being. Once you feel yourself in that space, formulate your intention. If you feel yourself as pain-free, then your intention can be to remain pain-free. If you feel yourself as flexible and mobile in your joints, your intention can be to have ongoing flexibility and mobility. If you feel into the space and feel young and invigorated, then incorporate this into your intention—to continue living with youth and vigor. Your intention can include all three of these feelings. Notice that I have used words like "remain, ongoing, continue." Project your intention into the future. Don't limit yourself to just tomorrow or the next week or even the next year.

Let the Big Guns Steer You

Another key to selecting a powerful intention is to stay in the feeling and not crowd the intention with "rules" you are holding.

What do I mean by this?

Just as you saw from the description of the assemblage point, the possibilities that exist in the Universe are vaster than we can see through our limited window. When your intention comes with specifics as to how things should turn out, the intention is limited and choked by your insistence that things go a certain way.

Let's use an example regarding knee pain. The intention "I intend that my right knee has no pain and that I can walk on the lake trail" is specific. You can see, however, how limited that intention is relative to "I intend that I walk easily and without pain." In the second instance, you are allowing Spirit/Universe/the Big Guns to steer you on a path that achieves more, applies to more situations, and considers more than just your knee.

Here is another example. Let's suppose that you were recently diagnosed with ovarian cancer. You are petrified, freaked out, and crying. All you can think of is how to hurry up and be cancer free. "I intend to be cancer-free" might be your initial intention. However, the typical path to arriving at a cancer-free place may be fraught with physical pain and distress from different types of chemotherapy and surgery, and you are still scared and crying. You may achieve cancer-free status, but will you have experienced a very enviable life on your way to getting what you intended? You may have days of suffering, of yourself and your family feeling stress, of having both physical and emotional complaints.

What if you were to let Spirit/Universe/Higher Self/Big Guns decide where you ultimately arrive and instead, focus your intention on having the best, most suffering-free, most vital life you can, both on the journey to conquer your cancer and beyond? What if you were to set the following intention: "I intend to bring all my resources to bear to bring about my most joyful, vibrant life"? Notice how in this second intention, you are seeing your life as extending beyond battling cancer, as including a calling in of all your spirit helpers and having a joyful life while getting to the place of no cancer.

Refocusing Based on Future Feelings

As we have talked about above, your intention is guided by your feelings. Using your imagination, you feel into your future self—how your body feels, the joy your heart feels, the future you are excited to be in. Sometimes, the path an intention leads to is not quite the desired one. In other words, you may not end up feeling exactly as you wanted.

Let's take knee pain as an example. Maybe you set your intention to be "I'll be pain-free," and you achieved a pain-free state, but you find you are still stiff and do not bend well, so your walking is limited. In other words, your intention did not bring about what you really wanted to feel beyond just being pain-free.

As you choose an intention, feel yourself into the new You that you are intending to experience. Is your intention sufficient? If you have learned that "pain-free" is not enough, you might now realize that what you really meant was that you wanted to be pain-free but also able to walk easily, with flexibility, and even able to hike.

As you "try on" each intention and consider it, if you find an intention lacking, refocus on your feeling state. Determine what you want to feel by seeing and feeling in your imagination the outcomes different intentions lead to. Use what you learn to refine and hone your intention.

In undergoing this process of discovering the right intention for yourself, it is as if you are imagining shooting one arrow and seeing that the target it hits isn't fully satisfying. Then you shoot another arrow toward a slightly different target, hit it, and realize that this target feels better for you. By refocusing your intention, you finally aim perfectly and land on the target that feels the best and is exactly what you wanted.

Note that creating the right intention does not have to be a long, involved process. On your first attempt, it may take you two or three refocused arrows to get to the right target, but as you practice feeling into who you will be and what you will experience in the future, the refining process will become second nature.

Affirmations

I want to briefly talk about affirmations, then we will do a journey to feel into the future You and flood your energy field with future, healed energy. Many people value the use of affirmations. In my experience, intentions are usually a more effective tool for transformation.

At first glance, affirmations sound a lot like intentions: "My body deserves to be healthy" or "I can heal myself" or perhaps "I take steps on my healing journey." Do you notice that there is a subtle but powerful difference between affirmations and intentions? Affirmations are statements that aim to bring about a feeling state in the here and now; intentions carry us to the future.

Using the phrase "I intend" will help direct your intention and remind you that you are looking ahead to the future. I find that the energetics of intentions are more powerful, because they engage your entire field and direct you to the future You.

One style of affirmation, however, is immensely powerful. An affirmation that begins with "I AM" floods your energy field with a cohesive energy, one that resonates with the power of Spirit in physical form. In religious scriptures, the words "I AM" were used by the writer at times when God appeared before humans. Thus, the use of I AM signifies high spiritual power. I AM statements that finish with positive endings, such as "cancer-free," pain-free," "long-lived," or "vibrant and healthy," are a strong addition to the other practices and techniques I have taught you.

The following meditative journey will help you visualize your future, healed self. You will notice that toward the end of the journey, you will be instructed to bring an image/feeling/state into your heart space. There are more complexities to this, but what you need to know is that, spiritually, many believe your heart space to be the center of your energetics, and connector between your soul and your physical form.

Meditation
Being the Future You

You will now embark on a meditative journey towards your healed, future self. Before you start, set your intention. Perhaps you set something like "I am healthy and vibrant" or "I intend that my health is free of limitations" or "I am vigorous, joyful, and alive." Remember: be in quiet space and open sacred space before journeying. When done, offer gratitude and close sacred space.
  Now, get comfortable, and let's begin.

[Start recording]

- Start by taking some nice, deep, relaxed breaths. In through your nose, and out through your mouth. Find yourself drifting deeper and deeper. Bring your awareness to your heart space. Take a few moments to connect with your energy field as you feel your heartbeat.

[Pause]

- Allow your breathing to slow down, as your entire awareness resonates with your heart space.

[Pause]

- Call in any spirit helpers you would like to join you on this journey. Feel the energy of your heart space change as they step in to join you.

[Pause]

- Now, move your awareness from your heart space, carrying yourself to a path in a location that makes you joyful and happy. It may be the beach or a mountain trail or a path through the woods. See it or sense it or just know it as your awareness arrives at this place.

[Pause]

- Feel the sun shining down on you as you walk along this path. Notice how good you feel on this path in this location. Take a few moments to stand in this beauty, sensing your energy field here.

[Pause]

- Now, shift your awareness to feel how you would like to feel in the future in your healed state. Take a few moments to truly connect with all you intend, and sense this good feeling flooding your heart space.

[Pause]

- Now, turn your awareness to the path in front of you. In the distance, you see a form walking toward you.

[Pause]

- As the form gets closer, you recognize that it is You, a healed You. Notice what aspects have shifted. Notice what color the healed You is, or any other special characteristics.

[Pause]

- Feel how vibrant and joyful the healed You is.

[Pause]

- The healed You approaches, and the two of you sit down together beside the path. You can feel how similar and close the two of you are. In fact, there is more in common between the two of you than you might have thought. You love the energy this healed You emits. Take a few moments to feel the healed You, all the energy and color and vibrancy.

[Pause]

- Imagine the energy of the healed state as a golden light. Allow this to wash over you, your energy field, your body, your soul.

[Pause]

- Now, ask the healed You if it will energetically join with you.

[Pause]

- Then, bring the image or sensation or knowing of the healed You into your field, anchoring it in your heart space. Take in the healed You, allowing it to spread from your heart space, percolating through your energy field, through your cellular machinery. Notice how you feel as the healed state becomes embodied internally.

[Pause]
- Take a few moments to integrate the healed state within you.

[Pause]
- Now, offer gratitude for all you have learned and all you have shifted. Commit to holding the image and feeling of this healed state within you, as you go forward in the following days and weeks. And now bring your awareness back to the current time and place. And open your eyes.

[Stop recording]

You may notice that the energetics of this journey are about visualizing the healed state, anchoring it firmly in your awareness, and then consciously integrating it into your field.

Whenever you create a journey, you also can make sure that you are guided from thought to energy field and then into your body. In this way, you will create a journey that encompasses similar energetics, to use as powerful tools to shift a health challenge.

Here is one last point about intentions: Be sure that in doing the work of finding just the right intention, you write it down—at least until you have more ease in thinking them up and holding them in your mind. You might even want to post the intention in a place in your home where you can see it often.

Once your intention is clear, it's time to do some shamanic rituals and use some energy techniques to energize and *Affirm* your newly shifted state. After all, you want your intention to be manifested in your life!

Affirm with Ritual

We are at the final step on our journey of Wheels. You have learned how to become more aware of your health issue and ways to discover hidden insights that can help you shift. You then tapped into the vast resources available to you, including higher vibrational energies of Nature and Spirit, to gain allies on your journey. You allowed these energetic allies to amplify your efforts to achieve healing, then you moved into formulating an intention, a most powerful act for connecting your desire to your thoughts, and sent that intention out into your energy field.

Now, you will step onto the part of the Wheel of Inner Actions where you will use rituals to lock in your intention, affirming your true desire to yourself and to Spirit.

I am introducing these rituals to you in an order that energetically feels correct to me. To start with, you'll want to connect with the Big Guns (Spirit, Nature, life force). Then, you'll clear away things that are causing your field, and hence your physicality, to be stagnant or blocked. You'll next bring in higher-vibrational, illuminated energies. Finally, you'll activate *ayni* (right relationship) by offering gratitude. You want to be allied with your spirit helpers when you undertake important sacred actions.

In all of these rituals, bear four important instructions in mind:

◊ First, work within sacred space so that you honor your allies in Spirit.

◊ Second, alter your consciousness so that you are not in ordinary awareness. You want to be able to tune into subtle energies and work with them. You've learned and practiced some simple ways to do that. The more ritualistic exercises in this chapter might be more challenging if you haven't done the basic shamanic exercises.

◊ And third, do *not* try to bring high-potency, high-vibrational life force into your body when there are ongoing errors in your field that have led to disorganized cellular machinery, such as cancer. In other words, you do not want to feed an imbalanced energy field; that just adds potency and power to the imbalance. Energetically, your field needs to be cleared first. It makes sense to always get connected and then do a clearing, so you have the best "soil" in which to "plant" the new energies. In fact, this book began with a journey to the Hall of Contracts to start your health shift with an intention and process to discard (clear) the rules under which you were operating and be ready to bring in a new paradigm.

◊ Finally, the fourth instruction to keep in mind is this: Perform a ritual of gratitude to respect the energies helping you.

Setting Up by Creating a Sacred Vortex and a Mesa (Medicine Bundle)

Along with creating an inner sacred space within which to work, as described in chapter 7, you might also find that having an altar, tabletop, or desktop on which to do energetic practices helps activate the sacred energy vortex in which you will do your work.

I sense a slight energetic difference between sacred space and a sacred energy vortex. Sacred space, to me, is more diffuse and exists around me as I am doing shamanic work. When I open my mesa (medicine bundle) and work with it, power builds over the cloth and around and within the sacred objects. This feels more focused and represents a channel between me and Spirit, so I call it a sacred vortex. The more often you engage in shamanic practices in this space, the greater the power that will build in the vortex.

You might also choose to create a mesa for yourself. A mesa is a sacred representation of you that consists of stones, crystals, feathers, and other talismans with which you form an alliance and which you will use in your practice. For example, to outline a "body proxy"—a figure representing your body that you will do shamanic work on so that your own body will experience the energetic effects.

To assemble a mesa, start by choosing a cloth that will serve as a wrap to protect the sacred tools you collect. Plan to have a minimum of seven stones or objects in your mesa, because you will use these with a body proxy to affect your chakras energetically. Over time, you will build an affinity with each stone. Before putting them into the mesa, each object should be cleared of any energies clinging to them. You can clear them by:

◊ passing it through a flame several times;

◊ spritzing it with sacred waters such as Florida water, flower water, or rosewater spray (you can find bottles of sacred water on websites that offer shamanic tools for sale);

◊ "smudging" it with the smoke of sacred incense (palo santo, copal, sage, sweetgrass, lavender, or similar);

◊ dipping it into a bowl of water that has a few drops of sacred essential oil (frankincense, juniper, rose, cedarwood).

Before starting your shamanic work, open your cloth and spread it out over the altar or tabletop, and when you are finished, wrap up your objects in the cloth. The very way you close your mesa holds ritualized energy, so be deliberate and sacred in the opening and closing of your mesa. The more time you spend with your mesa, the more time you are spending on your sacred inner work. As you move objects around in your mesa, as you open the cloth and spritz your stones, as you pray over your mesa, you are having conversations (however silent) with Spirit.

If you would like to learn more about the ways that the indigenous Q'ero of the Andes make and keep a mesa, you might want to connect with Wake Wheeler. A wise teacher who has also become my friend, Wake has studied the symbols and meanings of Q'ero mesa cloths and is a master at the rituals of the mesa as ancient indigenous people performed them.[24]

Talismans and objects that can assist in shamanic practices include stones, crystals, feathers, and more. Some people have small figurines of power animals or angels. I have a small black-green jade carving that I found in a Guatemalan village market that, to me, holds the power of man's connection to the land. Each object should be considered when you are in sacred space, to determine if it belongs in your mesa. Even if an object comes into your mesa now, it does not mean that it must stay with you. Remember: Your mesa is You. As you transform your inner and outer worlds, your mesa may change. As mentioned above, each object should be cleared before joining your mesa, and if you no longer feel affinity with an object, please release it outdoors to the earth with gratitude. Please do not throw the object into the trash.

As your mesa is a direct energetic connection to you and represents your growth and shifts, you should pay attention to and engage with your mesa. Connect with it in meditation or when you are in a prayerful state, expressing respect and gratitude. How would you do that, other than just saying the words over your mesa? The shamans of Peru describe the process of connection with gratitude as "feeding" your mesa. From time to time—daily or weekly—you should open your mesa and offer "energetic uplifts." By this I mean, spritz the contents of the mesa with sacred water, pass each object over the flame one by one, or hold each object over the smoke of incense or smudge. It is standard practice to not wash your mesa cloth, as the energies of your personal work have built up here. You may put the objects to the side and shake your cloth outdoors.

You can also bring in items of beauty to your mesa, such as flowers (dried or fresh), herbs (dried or fresh), or any items you consider representative of the beauty of Nature. I have brought in a pine cone I collected on a walk, a dried flower pod from my garden, and even kernels of dried heirloom Native American corn. The point is to honor your mesa.

When you are using fire (candle flame) to clear, be sure to have a candle that when lit can safely drip its wax into a saucer rather than onto your cloth. I personally like short, fat, votive-style candles rather than long tapers because when you are moving your hands in clearing practices and taking energies to the transformational flame, it is harder to move your hands from clearing energy at one level (usually a few inches off the cloth) up to the height of a long taper candle.

We will see in practices described below that you will use your hands to clear and smooth the energy field and then you will send the cleared energies to the flame by flicking your hands at the flame (with intention of transformation!). Perhaps you will use a feather (or a crystal or a stone) to "wipe" the energy field and then will pass the feather through the flame (quickly so you don't burn your feather!).

If you are unable to burn a candle, you can energetically wash energies off in another way. You can clear away energy and "discharge" the energies into a bowl of water that has a few drops of a sacred essential oil. When you are finished with your practice, carefully pour the water onto the land with the intention of sending energies to the earth to be transmuted. An unceremonious dumping of the water down the sink or the toilet won't do, it is important to hold the intention of the energies being transmuted.

Note: If you leave fresh flowers or herbs, be sure to check your mesa and remove them when they are wilted and possibly moldy. Dried ones can stay longer, but it is a good idea to change them out now and then.

Clearing Your Energy Using a Body Proxy and Your Mesa

You can clear your energy by using the exercise you learned in chapter 9, but once you have a mesa you can do a more complex ritual, using a modification of the basic method of clearing the energy field taught in the Four Winds training.

In the original practice, the client lies on their back while the shaman works in the energy field several inches above their body. Stagnant, blocked, or foreign energies are "found" (sensed, intuited, known) by the shaman, pulled out of the client's field, and passed to the flame to transmute. Then, high-vibrating, healing energy is brought into the field to fill in the empty spaces left by the removal of unwanted energies.

This cleansing is one you can do for yourself using a body proxy to stand in for your own body. In creating this proxy, I like to use seven stones, each representing a chakra. The first energy center of the body is between the legs, at the very base of the spine, also called the root chakra. Beneath the navel in the lower belly is the second chakra, or sacral chakra. Just under the ribs in the solar plexus, or upper belly, you find the third chakra. The heart holds the fourth chakra. The throat houses the fifth chakra. Between the eyebrows is the sixth chakra, also known as the third-eye chakra. At the top of the head is the seventh, or crown, chakra.

To work with a body proxy, place each of your seven stones so they mirror the arrangement of your body's chakras. Each of the chakras is associated with a color, starting with red (first chakra), followed by orange (second chakra), yellow (third chakra), green (fourth chakra), blue (fifth chakra), indigo (sixth chakra), and violet (seventh chakra). I love to use different colored stones to represent each of the seven centers. I have enjoyed collecting red jasper, carnelian, citrine, malachite, blue topaz, blue tourmaline, and amethyst to represent the chakra colors. You might find these stones at a store that sells crystals and other supplies for doing energy work, including shamanic practice. However, if you like, you can simply use seven stones or crystals. You will keep the objects in a mesa to prevent unwanted energies from attaching to them. Cleanse them before and after their use in creating a body proxy or for shamanic practices for healing.

I make a body proxy by imagining the client lying on the mesa cloth in front of me, on their back, head to my left. When you do this for yourself, place a stone at each of the (sensed) seven energy centers, or chakras. Alternately, you can forego the energy centers as markers for different places of the body and place a stone for each limb, one for the belly, one for the chest, one for the head—or any configuration that makes sense to you as you begin to do shamanic work with the body proxy.

In sacred space, with your mesa open and body proxy established, a lit candle at your side, place your hand over the body formed by mesa articles (holding a few inches above is good). When you sense energy that does not belong or that does not have enough flow of life force, move your hand in a counterclockwise manner, as if you are unwinding that area. As you'll remember from our discussion of medicine wheels, the correct flow of the energy field and chakras is clockwise. By moving your hand counterclockwise, you are removing any unwanted toxic energy you sense. Pull them out, tug on them, scrape them from the energy field, or dig them out—whatever you sense is the best way to remove these toxins. While doing this, hold a firm intention that you are clearing that which does not belong, that does not serve you. Place all the toxic energies into the flame to be transformed by the fire. Continue until you sense completion, working on more than one area of the body proxy if you sense blockages in more than one place.

When all of the energies that don't belong in the field are cleared from it, you're ready to bring in higher energies to fill the empty spots. With intention, raise your arms, palms open to the sky. Even if you are working indoors, intend to connect to the sky and the angelic realms. When you recognize that you have done so, gather high-level energy from above, bring it down and place it into the empty spots in the field over your body proxy.

To help you feel or sense that you are pulling in the energy, you might visualize that you are reaching up to a bucket of infinite golden light floating in the heavens above your head and tipping the bucket over slightly so that a stream of liquid gold, of amber light, pours down from the heavens into the field surrounding the body proxy and spilling into all the proxy. See, sense, know, or feel the golden light percolating through the whole body, bringing repair, restoration, and rejuvenation as it does its healing work.

Note: The light I describe is golden. That's because for me, golden light is very high-vibrational light. You may choose another color. Just be sure to sense that the color you are choosing has high-quality spiritual energy for healing.

Exercise

Doing a Focused Clearing

If you are having issues with a specific body area, you can do a focused clearing of your energy field. Ideally, choose an object from your mesa, because you have done sacred work using it, so it is building up healing powers. Intend that your object will assist in healing a specific area. For example, if you have chronic abdominal pain, find the place where the pain is worst.

- To begin, light a candle, and pass the object you will be using over the flame. Alternatively, you could spritz it with sacred water. Enter sacred space, and drop into relaxation, altering your consciousness through drumming, rattling, or other means. Then, use the feather or crystal to make counterclockwise circles directly over the actual physical area you wish to shift. After several circles, pass the object over the flame to release the extracted energies. Repeat the counterclockwise clearing several times until you sense the cleansing has been completed.

- Next, bring liquid golden light into that area, by raising your arms and drawing the light in from the sky. When you sense the area is saturated with the liquid gold, make focused clockwise circles over the specific area, sealing the healing energy into your body.

- Lastly, take the crystal or feather and wipe down your body from head to toe in sweeping motions, with the intention to smooth your energy field. You can wipe your head and face and then move to each arm, and then the chest and the back (using your intention as you won't be able to reach those areas with your hand motions). Finish with the belly and legs. See, sense, know, or feel your field restoring, just as you sensed this when working with the multicolored tapestry.

Exercise

Clearing Using "The River"

The River is another way to clear the energy field of stagnant or blocked energies using your mesa and sacred objects. Have a lit candle available, should you choose to use it. As always, work in sacred space, alter your consciousness, ask your helpers to be present, and finish with gratitude (and the closing of sacred space if you want to use an opening and closing ritual when doing this work). You may use the body proxy or any other representation of a path moving from left to right. I suggest you line up your stones as if marking a path that represents your life journey, flowing from left to right, from past to future.

- As you drop into relaxed awareness, set the intention to increase the flow of life force (the river) of your life. See (sense/visualize/ know/feel) where along the river your flow got blocked or diminished.

- Use your sensing to clear away any barriers, and use your hands to sweep energy from left to right, intensifying your river's force. You may see barriers as fallen trees clogging the river or as areas where muddy banks have eroded into the water, where debris has gathered damming up the flow.

- You may release those barriers to the flame to ensure the barriers stay gone. See places where your river escaped its banks, leading to a dissipation or weakening of the forward flow. Do what you need to do to remove barriers to your flow, to harness all your life force, to make your river strong and powerful as it moves into the future (on the right side of your mesa).

- Now sit with the newly cleaned, newly energized river. Take a few moments to pull into your deepest awareness and your energy field the improved forward motion of your life force, which you have been able to sense and affect.

Exercise

A Ritual to Eliminate the Negative (Symptoms of a Health Challenge)

This Eliminate the Negative ritual will help you get rid of distressing symptoms. You can do it using your mesa and sacred objects or without them, using a self-hypnosis practice.

To perform the ritual using your mesa, gather a few fresh flowers or dried flower petals, some incense (or a smudging stick, as described earlier), and some sacred water (again, as described earlier). Prepare yourself, your mesa, and sacred objects.

- Enter sacred space, and ask your spirit helpers to be present. Set the intention to reduce a distressing symptom, such as knee pain or headaches or shortness of breath. You may ask to reduce the activity of a tumor or heart disease or memory loss.

- Next, you will select stones to place in a group on your open mesa cloth. The number of stones should represent the level of distress of your symptom, so if you have seven stones, move over stones from your main group to represent where your symptom is. Perhaps your knee pain is a 7 out of 7 or your headache is a 6 out of 7. You may have collected and worked with more than seven stones. If so, just pull from your group of stones the number that represents your level of distress.

- Enter a state of deep awareness and then pass the smoke of incense or smudge stick over the stones or spritz them with sacred water. As you do this, hold your intention firmly. Reduce the magnitude of the distressing symptom or issue with intention and with your command, showing the shift by moving a stone out of the group when you discern that it is time to remove it.

- Set the stone aside. Sprinkle a few flower petals around the group of stones and the outlying stone, signifying the beauty of the inner work you are doing.

- Continue to hold your deep intention, removing one stone at a time, intuiting when it is appropriate to do, knowing that each time you remove a stone you are reducing the magnitude of the symptom or issue you're working to heal. Intermittently, sprinkle more flower petals, or smudge, or spritz. Continue removing stones one at a time, until you sense that you have removed what you intuit to be the appropriate number. You will know when to stop.

When your work is complete, sit in deep awareness and offer gratitude, knowing that you have made a powerful shift. If you did not move all the stones, you can always return to this practice. It may take several sessions to reduce the intensity of a symptom.

✿

Exercise
Dial It Up or Down

Another way to accomplish this energetic shift is to do this practice in a state of self-hypnosis. Work in sacred space, and record a script that leads you to deepen into relaxation and enter your heart space.

Ask your sacred helpers to be present for you, then focus your intention on reducing a symptom or health challenge. For example, perhaps you wish to diminish the tightness in your lower back and its lack of flexibility.

- To start, visualize yourself in a control room, directing all the activity of your body and energy field. As you look around the control room, see all the dials and gauges that represent functions of the body and energy field. Find the gauge that directs tightness in your back, if that's one of your symptoms. Perhaps it is a gauge that directs tightness of all muscles. Reach over and change the dial to reduce the tightness. Did you dial it down enough? If not, reach over and dial it down a little more. Find exactly where you want the setting of the dial to be, and move it to that place.

- Now look at the flexibility gauge. Set it exactly where you want it to be so that you can increase your flexibility, dialing it up as much as you desire.

- You choose any dial to represent control over any function. For example, you can dial down your gut distress, which occurs when you are eating out socially, or you can dial up your capacity for breath when exerting yourself. You can shut off the redness and pain from a bad sunburn, turning the dial to 0.

- When you have set the dials where you want them to be, offer gratitude to your spirit helpers for being present, leave the control room, and return to the current time and place. Close sacred space.

Getting Right with Spirit by Anchoring into Life Force

When I consider bringing healed, vibrant, and alive energy into the body, I energetically connect with and anchor to the life force. Life force is that which keeps you alive, your cellular machinery going, and your heart pumping. The quickest way I know to link with the life force is by connecting your heart space to the earth and stars.

The background assumptions of this practice are twofold. First, it's based on the idea that humans are intricately and perpetually linked to the earth (its molecules, minerals, and more) and to the galaxy. Second, life force flows from and is integral to this connection. This understanding is as simple as knowing that humans cannot exist without the earth, and the earth cannot exist without the galaxy and beyond.

Meditation

Earth Sky Heart

The following is a modified version of the Earth Sky Heart meditation taught by Drunvalo Melchizedek in his book *Living in the Heart: How to Enter Sacred Space within the Heart.*[25] You may record this script for yourself.

[Start recording]

- Go into sacred space, and quiet your awareness with your breath.

[Pause]

- Visualize bringing your awareness into the chest and into the back of the heart. Find the sacred space of the heart, and enter it. You know this space instinctively.

[Pause]

- Make your way into this sacred room, and take a seat. Observe the sacred room of your heart. Observe its details. Then, from the center of your sacred space of the heart, imagine a ball of golden light growing inside your heart.

[Pause]

- From that ball of golden light, send a beam of golden light down into the earth. Feel all the love you have for the earth. Feel it by remembering a beautiful sunset or field of wheat or bouquet of flowers. Send your love beaming from your heart space down the cord of golden light to the earth. Send the earth your love.

[Pause]

- Now, stop and feel the love coming back to you from the earth. Take in the love and connection from the earth. Feel the energy going down to the earth along the golden beam and back up to your heart. Feel the power of the life force and of this connection.

[Pause]

- Now, from the center of your heart, send a beam of golden light up to the heavens. Feel all the love you have for the sky beaming from your heart space to the heavens.

[Pause]

- Do this by remembering a gorgeous blue sky, the beauty of a starry night, or the full moon. Send your love to the sky. Now, stop and feel the love coming back to you from the sky. Take in the love and connection from the sky. Feel the energy going up to the sky along the golden beam and back down into your heart.

[Pause]

- Feel the power and life force of this connection.

[Pause]

- As you continue to feel yourself inside this golden column, also sense yourself inside this holy trinity of Earth, Sky, and Heart, and take in the life force this connection has. Drink in all that you need or want.

[Pause]

- The life force of the earth and sky is limitless. Through this vital connection, feel the restoration of your body, mind, and spirit.

[Stop recording]

Gratitude and Restoration of *Ayni* with a Despacho Ceremony

As I have said over and over throughout this book, staying in right relationship (*ayni*) with the forces and Spirit is critical to the future unfolding as you desire. A key shamanic ritual done by the Indians of the Andes is the despacho ceremony.

The despacho ceremony is often used by the Q'ero people of the Andes to offer prayers and offerings to Spirit. One at a time, participants add to a paper envelope or a cloth different items, such as candies, shells, ribbons, flowers, and leaves, which are symbols representing the natural world and its energies that accompany our prayers. Next, the items are prayed over, and the bundle is wrapped up and burned or buried. (Alberto Villoldo describes how to perform a despacho ceremony in his fourwinds.com blog.)[26] The ceremony is one of gratitude, our prayers and symbols of abundance, to Spirit. To perform one of these ceremonies is deeply moving and personally nurturing.

The ritual I offer here is a more simplified version that can be done indoors or outdoors. In the traditional ceremony, the prayer bundle is wrapped and burned or buried, a way to release the energies to Spirit and the Universe. In my version, the prayer offerings can be dismantled later and the ingredients dispersed in Nature or left outdoors to naturally dissipate over time.

Since you are embarking on a healing journey, your despacho (prayer bundle) will be a form of prayers to Spirit about your healing. To invoke this, you offer a despacho to Spirit, showing gratitude for what has happened and what will happen in your journey. Also, a despacho is recognition of your place in the cosmos—one with Nature, one with Spirit, one with *ayni,* or right relationship. Your intention during the making of this despacho is to refresh the relationship.

Gather items that offer joy and beauty and sweetness to provide nourishment to the earth. These items might be fresh flowers, small bits of chocolate or other candy, granulated sugar, dried herbs, dried seed pods, dried pieces of heirloom or ornamental corn, small pine cones, dried sage or lavender leaves, or pieces of beautiful ribbon or yarn. You might include rice or quinoa or small dried beans. Also, consider having available floral water sprays, such as rose or juniper water, or a small amount of an alcoholic beverage to spritz or splash over the prayer bundle. Over the years, I have purchased some dried herbs and flowers (lavender, jasmine, rosehips, saffron, calendula), and then have kept a bin of despacho ingredients to use later in future ceremonies.

If you are working outside, plan to leave your despacho in Nature—and make sure that the ingredients are all biodegradable (such as seeds and dried flowers). You would not want to leave a piece of ribbon or paper outdoors. If you are out walking or hiking and choose to stop and make a despacho, your ingredients would be those readily found around you, so candies, flowers, rice, ribbons, and so forth would not be part of this *au naturel* despacho. The essential component to your despacho is your presence, your intention, and your prayers and gratitude.

The basic ingredient in the indigenous Andean tradition is the use of a grouping of three coca leaves (called kintus). For your despacho, you can use dried bay leaves or leaves found outdoors. When working inside, start with a large piece of paper to make into an envelope to hold all the nourishing items. A cut-open paper bag will do. Spread that out on your mesa cloth. If you're outdoors, you will place the items or ingredients on the ground.

◊ First, hold a group of three leaves, or kintus, in your fingers, and with intention, blow your prayers and gratitude into the leaves. Then place them on the paper or the ground, arranging them intuitively. Continue placing the kintus, forming a circle as you lay them down in a clockwise manner in lines within a circle like the spokes of a wheel.

◊ Add other ingredients on top of the kintus, placing or dropping them in a clockwise manner. When you add flowers, you might remove some or all of the petals before sprinkling them over the other ingredients. You also might encircle the small mountain of ingredients with a piece of yarn or ribbon. (Petals are easily pulled from carnations.)

◊ You might then spritz the bundle with sacred water. In the traditional despacho, a flower (usually a carnation) is dipped into a small glass of wine and then shaken over the bundle, the drops of wine falling onto the other despacho items, before being laid on top of the bundle. The glass of remaining wine is poured out on the earth as an offering.

◊ When you are finished with your indoor despacho, wrap the large paper around the bundle, and tie it with a piece of ribbon or yarn. Later, go to a place in Nature and open the bundle, releasing the ingredients to Nature, then turn and walk away. It is customary to burn or bury the despacho, as you do not spend time with the bundle once it is offered; however, by simply leaving the ingredients in Nature, this conveys to Spirit and the earth that you are releasing any attachment to your desired outcome.

The Sand Painting

An oft-used practice in modern-day shamanic work is the practice of sand painting. Sand paintings were originally made by Native Americans, such as the Navajo (Diné) in the Southwest, and included bits of colored stone placed on a background of dry sand, representing gods, animals, or natural forces. Sand paintings also were used in healing ceremonies where the patient would sit in the center of the painting. Upon completion of the painting, which also incorporated applying pigment and sand on the patient, it would be destroyed, as all is changeable, nothing fixed.

In modern-day ceremonies, a sand painting is made in Nature, using natural materials, to symbolize the journey the person is on. Moving materials around the painting signify the changes the person wants to occur. In other words, the painting is a representation of or proxy for the inner world of the person. Any changes made to it can affect the individual's energy field.

The following practice is my variation of the sand painting, which I combine with elements of the despacho This practice is done outdoors, using elements of Nature.

○

Exercise
A Sand Painting Practice

- Go somewhere in Nature that feels good to you. Begin to collect items (sticks, pine cones, flowers, found objects) and, with intention, place these items in a pattern (drawing) that represents where you are on your healing journey. Make boundaries around the items to distinguish the group of items that represents you. Perhaps you still feel a bit congested physically with pain or a distressing symptom. Your painting might have a jumble of twigs in the center, and perhaps not feel as beautiful as you would like. With the intention of making inner shifts into the You that you want to be, move the objects within the painting, add new items, and "paint" yourself as you would like to be.

- The next step is to offer deep gratitude to Spirit for the shifts that are, and will be, happening. Have several items of beauty to offer the painting: a speckled stone, a dried blade of grass with a unique color, anything you choose. Imprint these offerings with your essence by using your intention to breathe your power into each item three times. Add your gratitude for the sacred process that is happening energetically as you do the painting and intend the inner shifts.

- Leave the painting overnight, and dismantle it the next day to indicate that you are turning the process and your desire over to Spirit. If you are unable to return to that spot in Nature the next day, hold an intention that the forces of Nature will shift the painting and do the surrendering for you.

The practices you have learned in this chapter evoke the fundamental energetics to *Affirm with Ritual* all the work you have done (*Aware, Allow, Act*) up until this point. You may have noticed that the distinction between the steps is not rigid; there is a lot of fluidity and blending between one step and another. Eventually, as you get more practice at working with shamanic healing techniques, many if not all these phases will occur simultaneously. You will become adept at using your intention to drive changes in your health challenge or challenges, and you will become fluent in understanding, at an instinctual level, that you should clear unwanted energies before you bring in greater life force.

Should you struggle with a particularly complex issue, you may need help from a seasoned shamanic practitioner. At the end of this book, you will find contact information for some of the shamanic healers I know and trust; also some shamanic and energy healing schools.

In the next and final chapter, I go through a few common ailments that I see in my medical practice and offer you ideas for shifting them. With more experience, you will see that my approach is not the only one and may not be how you would work. To this I say, "Wonderful!" You are healing yourself and know what you need and what works for you. That is what I have wished for. I send you my deepest intention for your health shift, my deepest gratitude for you taking the time to learn from me, and my fervent wish that you step into the Maximum You that I know you can be. Blessings on your journeys.

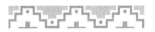

The Maximum Medicine
Approach to Common
Health Challenges

In this chapter, you'll learn about a few common issues I see in my medical clinic and how I might put together an approach to healing, using the techniques and practices I described in previous chapters. There are a few important caveats that we need to handle first, however.

First, it may take you a while to get these practices under your belt, so even if you are frustrated with the state of Western medicine, don't hesitate to seek traditional Western medical help for your illness or symptoms of a health condition. If you're experiencing anything truly urgent—you have a fever or a lump that has been growing, you're passing out or having bad pain, you're unable to breathe easily—it's even more important that you see a physician. You can use shamanic techniques as adjuncts while you are undergoing traditional treatment for any condition, keeping in mind that it's safest to do clearing before bringing in healing energy.

Second, do not stop any of your prescribed medications without discussing it with your physician. Yes, you can shift blood pressure and diabetes with shamanic techniques; however, please have a conversation with and maintain oversight by your physician as you use other approaches to make shifts. In other words, do not make an either/or decision about your approach to healing. Blending styles offers a lot of breadth and depth.

Let me be clear: I want you to be safe. It makes no sense to suffer through a bad strep throat or worse while you are learning shamanic practices. You may need the help of a Western medicine physician at times.

I am going to tell you about some of the topics I think about as a Western medicine physician dealing with patients who have common health challenges, and I'll discuss approaches you can use to bring in a blend of shamanic and energy practices. It's important to remember that when you use shamanic practices, it's essential to work in sacred space, ask for the presence of your spirit helpers when needed, and practice *ayni* (right relationship) by closing sacred space with gratitude, as you've learned in this book.

My approaches are not perfect. If your intuition guides you to some other intervention (for example, acupuncture or a particular energy medicine approach, such as Healing Touch), please, of course, follow your intuition. After all, that is what you are growing now, so use it.

Also, I strongly encourage you to remember the journey of the Chacana and to work with the five medicine wheels we discussed in detail in this book. Open your awareness and use your intuition to get clarity on how to proceed. Ask for and allow your spirit helpers to amplify your power. Set an intention, plan your actions, then anchor in and affirm the energetic changes you would like to experience, using rituals and making lifestyle changes. Healing awaits!

At the end of this chapter, you'll find an invocation or prayer I have created for you as you undertake your personal journey to shift a health challenge. Surrounded and assisted by my own spirit helpers, I have infused this invocation with my strong intention for your healing. The prayer is encoded for your success.

In the references section at the end of this book, I offer resources you can use to help with your health challenge. You may find that you make better headway when an energy or shamanic healer works with you early on and jumpstarts things, rather than working alone. The groups and practitioners I have listed are people whom I would trust with my own health.

Anxiety and Depression

All of us struggle with worries and sadness at some point in our lives. Some of us struggle with these emotions on a day-to-day, chronic basis. Unfortunately, more of us are struggling with anxiety and depression than ever due to what is going on in the world.

Seek traditional medical care if you are feeling that you want to die, have a plan to hurt yourself, are thinking of hurting others, or are experiencing abnormal thoughts, such as hallucinations and paranoia. These thoughts mean something is very wrong with your brain chemistry, and that situation should be addressed immediately by a physician, even if it means going to an emergency room or calling a crisis hotline.

When I am wearing my traditional Western medicine hat, I think about the following when talking with a person who is feeling very sad and/or anxious:

◊ Are they drinking too much caffeine or using too many stimulants?

◊ Are they using other mind-altering substances?

◊ Do they possibly have a metabolic abnormality, such as a vitamin deficiency or thyroid disease?

◊ Do they have an abnormality in their brain physiology, such as history of a stroke or tumor?

◊ Is their diet imbalanced?

◊ Are they getting outdoors enough?

◊ Are they getting enough exercise?

◊ Are they getting enough good quality sleep?

◊ Is there a relationship that is putting significant stress on them?

◊ Is there any abuse or trauma involved?

◊ Do they demonstrate any underlying loss of mental capacity, such as dementia?

◊ Are they mentally capable of engaging in therapy and capable of taking their medications if they are prescribed any?

◊ Do they have a good support system to help them cope while the medications I prescribe are kicking in?

Here are some considerations for shamanic and energetic practices:

◊ Spend more time outside in Nature, and in particular, get enough sunlight. Experiencing sunlight generates life force.

◊ Consciously connect to the earth and sky. The more this connection is strengthened, the more a part of this great trinity you will feel. It is hard to be anxious or sad when you are deeply connected to the earth and sky. You begin to remember your true and grander essence and purpose—in other words, you get over\your literal-world, human self.

The earth draws off excess, short-circuiting energy from your field. Try lying on a beach or in a meadow or a grassy backyard, and look up at the sky and any clouds for a few minutes and see how you feel.

◊ Meditate or pray with Spirit, or perform a ritual to connect you to Spirit. In this book, you've learned about several ways to connect, but you might intuit other ways that work for you.

◊ Think about whether anything needs to change in your diet, daily habits, exercise, or relationships. Dialogue with your Higher Self or the Wise One to learn more.

◊ Contemplate the source of your worries. Ask Spirit and your spirit helpers how you can de-escalate your worries or remove them completely. You can use the shamanic journey to the Hall of Contracts to learn about any contracts that are causing you to make a habit of unproductive worrying.

◊ Journey to the Control Room, and see yourself dialing down the panic or unplugging the control box for your worries.

◊ Write a relaxation script, using words such as "Allow yourself to relax deeper and deeper" or "Let all your worries drift away, leaving you calm and peaceful." Record the script, and play it several times during the day and before bed. You can also listen to audio recordings of relaxing meditations that others have recorded.

◊ Perform a clearing of your energy field, as described earlier in this book. Focus on the part of your body that feels your tension. Remove the anxious feelings, and release them to the flame of a candle. Afterward, if you work with a crystal as a cleansing tool, be sure to pass the crystal through a flame or spritz it with sacred water so that any harmful energies clinging to it will be removed.

◊ Make a prayer bundle, as described earlier, to express gratitude for you being able to live worry- and sadness-free—an intention you should set before doing this ritual. When performing it, pray as if you are already freed of the burden of modern-day worries.

COVID and Other Bacterial and Viral Illnesses

Traditional Western medicine's approach to these illnesses, which is a valuable one, is to explore:

◊ How sick is the patient?

◊ Is their breathing compromised?

◊ Do they have a high fever or abnormal heart rate?

◊ Are they taking in enough fluids? Is there risk of dehydration?

◊ Do they have other medical illnesses that complicate their ability to fight this infection?

◊ Do they need antiviral or antibiotic medications?

◊ Are they financially able to take off work to recuperate?

You can add a shamanic approach to dealing with any of these illnesses:

◊ Meditate or journey to get clarity on what diet/ herbal teas/immune-boosting foods would help and how best to recuperate. I am constantly surprised by how patients resist staying home and resting. Rest and sleep are very restorative.

◊ Do a cleansing to extract a foreign energy (bacteria/virus) from you. Set your intention to use crystals or a sacred object to remove this cause of illness. Smooth out your field after removal is done.

◊ Set a strong intention to receive help, form an alliance with high-vibration, high-power energy beings that can infuse your system with life force, restoring your body and its immune function. In sacred space, in prayerful mode, ask to connect with the highest-order energy, then intuitively bring that energy into your field. Remember to clear your luminous energy field before bringing in elevated, high-power energy.

◊ Dialogue with a Wise One (see chapter 4) to learn how you can best build and support your immune function on a daily, maintenance basis. This step is best done when you are recovering or recovered.

Gut Distress

Traditional Western medicine asks:

◊ Is this issue chronic or acute?

◊ Does something have to be done urgently? For example, should special X-rays be ordered, or should the stool be checked for pathologic bacteria and parasites?

◊ Is there diarrhea with blood?

◊ Is there weight loss or weight gain?

◊ If there's belly pain, is it focused in one place, or is it a diffuse, uncomfortable feeling?

◊ Does the distress happen in certain situations or when certain foods are eaten, such as milk? (Note: The three preceding questions are not routinely asked by Western medicine physicians; however, a functional medicine physician or dietician or nutritionist might ask them, so I've included them here. You might wish to add these professionals to your health care team.)

◊ How much soda and/or artificial sweetener is being consumed?

◊ What is the diet like? Is the patient eating enough fiber? (I had one patient who had *never in her life* eaten anything green. For years, her entire diet had consisted of fast foods like hot dogs and potato chips. Since that time, when I ask patients if they eat a balanced diet, I get them to walk me through what they eat on a typical day. In other words, I'll say, "Tell me what you ate for breakfast yesterday and then what did you have for lunch?" So many surprising details emerge when I take the time to do this.)

A shamanic approach to gut issues might include the following:

◊ A calming meditation using these words: *With each breath, I feel life force moving into and then out of my belly. I feel all my distress leaving with each exhale.*

◊ A journey into your belly and its wisdom. Engage in a dialogue with the part of you that governs your distress, asking for its help. For example, you could ask it why you get cramps or feel gassy or need to rush to the bathroom often. In your dialogue, be sure to ask what needs to change. For example, what do you need to stop doing or consuming? What do you need to do more of or bring in so that you can start to get relief and even healing? You might ask if there are foods you need to avoid and foods you need to eat more often. You can also ask your belly about situations that typically cause you gut distress. Intuit how you should minimize or remove yourself from these situations or people.

◊ A meditation on the Multicolored Light Tapestry of your personal energy field, as described earlier. Check for any attached energies that do not belong, and remove them, sending them into the flame of a candle for transformation. Check that the weave of the tapestry that is your luminous energy field is unbroken and flows smoothly around your physical body. Spend some time smoothing out and repairing your field. Finish restoring your energy field by "Running the Colors."

Joint and Back Pain

Traditional Western medicine's approach is to look at the following:

◊ Is the joint pain affecting one joint or many? (If it's many, that implies a systemic inflammatory process.)

◊ Are the joints red, hot, or swollen? (This implies a more serious inflammatory process.)

◊ Has there been a recent infection where the joints are red and hot? Has there been a recent fever or IV drug use, which can cause an infection?

◊ Did the joint or back pain start with an injury?

◊ Is the back pain accompanied by pain or jagging down a leg? (This would indicate a pinched nerve.)

◊ Has the patient complaining of back pain recently had prostate or breast cancer? (When these cancers metastasize, they go into the bone, which may cause back pain.)

◊ Is the pain so debilitating that the person needs to have blood tests or X-rays or see a specialist immediately?

Shamanic practices for treating joint or back pain could include:

◊ Connecting with a power animal or a celestial being, using the scripts suggested in this book.

◊ Intending to call upon a spiritual helper to help shift your joint pain. Meditate and dialogue with your spiritual helpers to access assistance in resolving your joint pain. During your dialogue, you can ask what dietary and lifestyle changes you should make. Do you need more of a specific element (Earth, Air, Fire, Water)?

◊ Getting into a meditative state and asking Spirit and any spirit helpers what you are holding onto in your skeleton that can be released. This may be the memory of an old trauma or emotional wound or it may be a contract you are operating under. Once you know it's there, you can address it energetically—for example, through a cleansing of your energy field or through a journey to the Hall of Contracts to rewrite the "rules" you are operating under/stuck with.

◊ Meditating and then journeying to your heart space or the Control Room so you can experience healing processes. Dialoguing with your spirit helpers may have suggested what needs healing.

◊ Perhaps imagining a soothing waterfall that washes away your pain and loss of mobility.

◊ Bringing in a power animal or spiritual helper to move through your field and search for and remove anything that is not in right order. You do this by meditating and calling on this entity to help you with this specific task. Have your helper carry the abnormalities away to a chamber with a sacred fire, or something symbolically similar. Remember: If you create a script for a journey or guided visualization, you'll want to use the elements I outlined earlier, including repetitive language that helps you go deeper into a meditative state, where you are more open to suggestion.

What follows next is my prayer for your healing. I have created this invocation with my deepest intent, that I offer with an open heart. in sacred space, with my spirit helpers gathered around. You may want to read this prayer before you embark on any of the exercises in this book and then use it over and over. It is more powerful if you speak it aloud.

Prayer

Invocation for Your Journey

I call to the power of the Four Directions—South, West, North, and East, and the forces of Nature associated with them—to come join me in summoning the most powerful and successful healing vortex.

I call to the power of the Elements—Fire, Water, Earth, and Air—to come bring the magic of their mysteries into the healing vortex.

I call to the power of the holy trinity of Earth, Human, and Sky to infuse this vortex with correct alignment and function of the human body.

I call to all spirit helpers, from earthbound elementals to celestial angelic beings, to bring forth the substantial and significant power of life force into this healing vortex.

I summon the protectors of this space, to guard and guide any healing work that occurs within this vortex.

I ask that anyone, myself included, who enters this vortex, while true of heart and intention, be gifted the mystery, magic, speed, and power of any and all healing that is available.

I ask that anyone who enters, myself included, whose desire is heartfelt, find release from any suffering of body, mind, and spirit.

I bow my head in reverence for the assistance brought, and, as always, I remain deeply grateful.

Thank you for your presence and guidance.

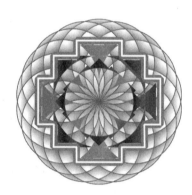

Afterword

What comes next after you have read this book and done all the practices? How should you go forward? You have seen how to look inward as well as out past your usual assemblage point and now have new, empowered perspectives. You have embodied the energies of wisdom, clarity, expansion, transformation, and more. You have journeyed to sacred places, both inside and outside of you, and each day you renew your relationship with your spirit helpers and with Heaven and Earth you are building your personal power and bringing more of You to your life and the world.

What does it mean to have a bigger, better You stepping into the world? On a global scale, your expanded capabilities are in sacred relationship with each other and the divine forces. Consequently, you will bring more awakening to our collective challenges and, therefore, more potential solutions, and that is a very good thing, for you and for all of us.

On an individual level you can rest easier, knowing that each time a challenge presents itself, you are now equipped to drill down to the place where you can steer the outcome. Whether that challenge is a health challenge or a life challenge, the same approach fits: Remember to practice the Four 'A's—be aware, allow help, choose an action, and affirm your choice daily.

With your new awarenesses, you can influence the health care system—both the people around you who may be patients, and the medical professionals you encounter who may be too resigned to how things are. You can steer those encounters in a new direction and, in doing so, help shift a broken system by bridging glorious mainstream science with the deep wisdom of our ancestors.

Join me. Restore the belief that each patient has immense power, particularly when in alliance with Earth and Spirit. Restore yourself, restore your community, restore our world. I bow to you with deep gratitude for the energy you are bringing and will bring into the world.

¡Salud!

Medicine Wheels and Chacana

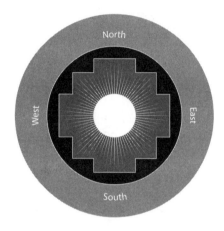

The Four Directions

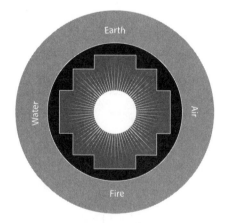

The Four Elements

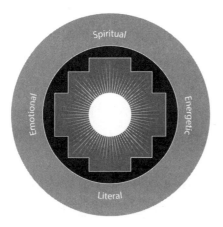

The Four Perspectives

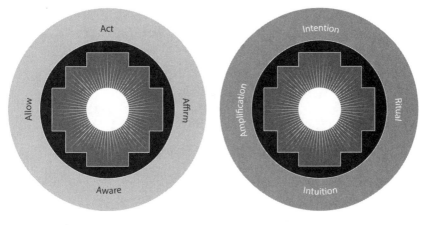

The Four Inner Tasks   The Four Inner Actions

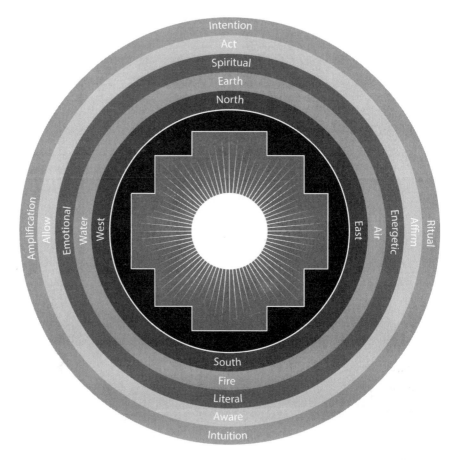

Combining the Five Medicine Wheels

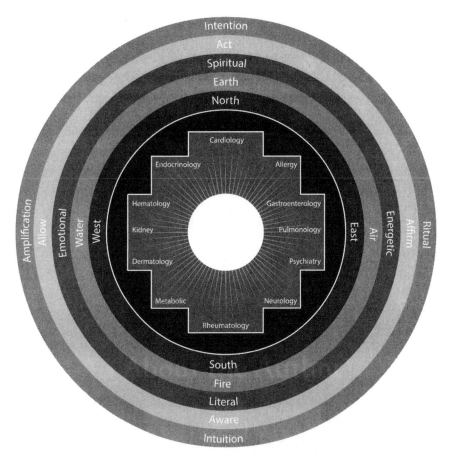

Combining Physiology with the Chacana
and the Medicine Wheels

Notes

[1] Information on the luminous energy field paraphrased from Dr. Alberto Villoldo, in my training with him, and on his website article "The Luminous Energy Field." https://thefourwinds.com/luminous-energy-field/

[2] K. C. Krycka, "Shamanic Practices and the Treatment of Life-Threatening Medical Conditions." *Journal of Transpersonal Psychology*, 2000: 32(1), 69–87.

[3] Nicholas Bakalar, "The Alternative Medical Bill: $30.2 Billion," *New York Times*, June 27, 2016.

[4] Lynne McTaggart, *The Field: The Quest for the Secret Force of the Universe*, Updated ed. (New York: Harper Perennial, 2008).

[5] Thomas E. Mails, *Fools Crow: Wisdom and Power* (Tulsa, OK: Council Oak Books, 2001), 128–130.

[6] Mails, *Fools Crow*, 149.

[7] Richard Gerber, M.D., *Vibrational Medicine: The #1 Handbook of Subtle-Energy Therapies*, 3rd edition. (Rochester, VT: Bear & Company, 2001).

[8] Anodea Judith, *Charge and the Energy Body: Your Vital Key to Healing Your Life, Your Chakras, and Your Relationships* (Carlsbad, CA: Hay House, 2018).

[9] Carolyn McMakin, *The Resonance Effect: How Frequency Specific Microcurrent Is Changing Medicine*, (Berkeley, CA: North Atlantic Books, 2017), 99–104.

[10] Danielle MacKinnon, *Soul Contracts: Find Harmony and Unlock Your Brilliance* (New York: Atria Publishing and Beyond Words, 2014).

[11] Michael Newton, *Journey of Souls: Case Studies of Life Between Lives*, (Woodbury, MN: Llewellyn Publications, 2010).

[12] Carl Greer, Ph.D., Psy.D., *Change Your Story, Change Your Life: Using Jungian and Shamanic Tools to Achieve Personal Transformation*, (Scotland: Findhorn Press, 2014), 106–108.

[13] Rita Faith and Neville Goddard, *Master Your Inner Game to Achieve Your Every Desire: Book 1 Inner Talking*, (CreateSpace Independent Publishing Platform, 2016). The first quotation is from the book's introduction; the second is from its back cover.

[14] Barbara Brennan, *Hands of Light: A Guide to Healing Through the Human Energy Field* (New York: Bantam Press, 1988).

[15] Dawson Church, *Mind to Matter: The Astonishing Science of How Your Brain Creates Reality* (Carlsbad, CA: Hay House, 2019), 150.

[16] David Hawkins, *The Map of Consciousness Explained: A Proven Energy Scale to Actualize Your Ultimate Potential* (Carlsbad, CA: Hay House, 2020).

[17] Don Miguel Ruiz, *The Four Agreements: A Practical Guide to Personal Freedom* (San Rafael, CA: Amber-Allen Publishing, Inc., 1997).

[18] Carlos Castaneda, *Power of Silence: Further Lessons from Don Juan*, original edition (New York: Washington Square Press, 1991).

[19] Jaap van Etten, *Dragons: Guardians of Creative Powers* (Flagstaff, AZ: Light Technology Publishing, 2019).

[20] Ted Andrews, *Animal Speak: The Spiritual & Magical Powers of Creatures Great and Small* (Woodbury, MN: Llewellyn Publications, 2002), 1.

[21] Diana Cooper, *Dragons: Your Celestial Guardians* (Carlsbad, CA: Hay House UK, 2018), 3.

[22] Oxford Language Dictionary Online.

[23] Esther Hicks and Jerry Hicks. *The Amazing Power of Deliberate Intent: Living the Art of Allowing* (Carlsbad, CA: Hay House, Inc. 2007).

[24] Wake Wheeler, https://www.sacredpathways.us

[25] Drunvalo Melchizedek, *Living in the Heart: How to Enter Sacred Space within the Heart* (Flagstaff, AZ: Light Technology Publishing. 2003), 128–130.

[26] Alberto Villoldo, "What Is a Despacho?" April 26, 2016. https://thefourwinds.com/blog/shamanism/what-is-a-despacho/April 26 2016.

Bibliography

Books

Andrews, Ted. *Animal Speak: The Spiritual & Magical Powers of Creatures Great and Small*. Woodbury, MN: Llewellyn Publications, 2002.

Brennan, Barbara. *Hands of Light: A Guide to Healing Through the Human Energy Field*. New York: Bantam Press, 1988.

Castaneda, Carlos. *Power of Silence: Further Lessons from Don Juan*. New York: Washington Square Press/Simon and Schuster, 1991.

Cavendish, Richard, ed. *Man, Myth and Magic – Volume 19*. New York: Marshall Cavendish, 1970.

Church, Dawson. Mind to Matter. Carlsbad, CA: Hay House, 2018.

Cooper, Diana. *Dragons: Your Celestial Guardians*. London: Hay House UK, 2018.

Faith, Rita, and **Neville Goddard**. *Master Your Inner Game to Achieve Your Every Desire: Book 1 Inner Talking*, CreateSpace Independent Publishing Platform, 2016.

Gerber, Richard. *Vibrational Medicine. The #1 Handbook of Subtle Energy Therapies*. Rochester, VT: Bear & Company/Inner Traditions, 2001.

Greer, Carl. *Change Your Story, Change Your Life: Using Shamanic and Jungian Tools to Achieve Personal Transformation*. Forres, Scotland: Findhorn Press, 2014.

Hawkins, David. *The Map of Consciousness Explained: A Proven Energy Scale to Actualize Your Ultimate Potential.* Carlsbad, CA: Hay House, 2020.

Hicks, Esther and **Hicks, Jerry**. *The Amazing Power of Deliberate Intent: Living the Art of Allowing.* Carlsbad, CA: Hay House, 2007.

Judith, Anodea. *Charge and the Body: Your Vital Key to Healing Your Life, Your Chakras, and Your Relationships.* Carlsbad, CA: Hay House, 2018.

Lipton, Bruce. *The Biology of Belief 10th Anniversary Edition: Unleashing the Power of Consciousness, Matter, and Miracles.* Carlsbad, CA: Hay House, 2016.

MacKinnon, Danielle. *Soul Contracts: Find Harmony and Unlock Your Brilliance. Illustrated edition.* Hillsboro, OR: Beyond Words, 2014.

Mails, Thomas. *Fools Crow: Wisdom and Power.* San Francisco, CA: Council Oak Books, 1991.

McMakin, Carolyn. *The Resonance Effect: How Frequency Specific Microcurrent is Changing Medicine.* Berkeley, CA: North Atlantic Books, 2017.

McTaggart, Lynne. *The Field: The Quest for the Secret Force of the Universe. Updated edition.* New York: Harper Perennial, 2008.

Melchizedek, Drunvalo. *Living in the Heart: How to Enter into the Sacred Space within the Heart.* Flagstaff, AZ: Light Technology Publishing. 2003.

Newton, Michael. *Journey of Souls: Case Studies of Life Between Lives.* Woodbury, MN: Llewellyn Publications, 2010.

Ruiz, Don Miguel. *The Four Agreements: A Practical Guide to Personal Freedom.* San Rafael, CA: Amber-Allen Publishing, 1997.

Van Etten, Jaap. *Dragons: Guardians of Creative Powers*. Flagstaff, AZ: Light Technology Publishing, 2019.

Online Sources

Bakalar, Nicholas. "The Alternative Medical Bill: $30.2 Billion." New York Times, June 27, 2016. https://www.nytimes.com/2016/06/28/health/alternative-complementary-medicine-costs.html.

Krycka, K. C. "Shamanic Practices and the Treatment of Life-Threatening Medical Conditions." Journal of Transpersonal Psychology, 32(1), 69–87, 2000.

Villoldo, Alberto. "The Luminous Energy Field." https://thefourwinds.com/luminous-energy-field)

Villoldo, Alberto. "What Is a Despacho?" April 26, 2016. https://thefourwinds.com/blog/shamanism/what-is-a-despacho/April 26 2016.

Wheeler, Wake. https://www.sacredpathways.us

Resources

Practitioners

If you're seeking help with healing, you might want to consider one of these talented shamanic practitioners whom I know personally:

Alison Normore, Ph.D. https://www.alisonnormore.com/. Alison is a true shaman sister. We trained in the Four Winds Light Body curriculum together. She carries on the teachings of Alberto Villoldo and mixes in her connections to the ancestors in her classes and healing work.

CC Treadway. https://www.lightschoolarts.com/. CC is a multifaceted person who has incredible capacities as an artist, musician, and energy worker. She also is a powerful channeler of messages from Spirit.

Lizzie Rose Reiss. https://www.magicisreal.org/. Lizzie is an energy worker and reiki practitioner who is deeply tapped into the realms of wonder, surprise, and magic.

Wake and Kinlen Wheeler. https://www.sacredpathways.us/. Wake and Kinlen are graduates of the Four Winds school and carry on their healing work and teachings following the indigenous traditions of the Andes.

Victoria Johnson. https://www.condorjourney.com/. Victoria is a classmate of mine from The Four Winds. She does shamanic healing and teaches students how to reclaim their life purpose.

Chris Waters. https://www.spiritoftheinca.com/. Chris is a classmate of mine from the Four Winds. She has continued her healing work as a shaman and coaches others to achieve life fulfillment.

Energy Medicine and Shamanic Schools

Barbara Brennan School of Healing:
https://barbarabrennan.com/find-healing-practitioner/

Donna Eden School of Energy Medicine:
https://practitioner.edenmethod.com/

The Four Winds Society:
https://thefourwinds.com/resources/

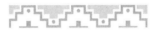

Index

Act, 82–84, 87–88, 92, 152
Affirm, 82–84, 87–88, 90
affirmations, 160
allies, 48, 56–57, 85, 105, 107, 128, 139, 143, 148, 156, 164
Allow, 82–84, 86–88, 90, 137
amplification, 84–87, 90, 137
ancestor, 41, 67, 93, 139
anxiety/depression, 182
assemblage point, 110–101, 158
Aware, 82–84, 86–88, 90
Ayni, 56, 58, 69, 75, 104, 108, 153, 164, 176–77, 182

back pain, 31, 54–58, 75, 101–102, 109, 111, 187–88

chacana, 63–65, 68, 81–82, 90–92, 94, 182, 193–96
chakras, 43, 46, 165, 168–69
clarity, 99, 101
communication, 99
consciousness, 40, 44, 47, 49, 53, 95–97, 99, 170–71, 198–99,
contract, 54–55, 58–62, 165, 184, 188
Crow, Frank Fools, 43– 44, 97

dialogue, 57–58, 61, 106, 129–30, 147, 184–85, 188

energy medicine, 13, 22, 27, 40, 43, 45–48, 55, 62–63, 182

excellence, 98–99, 102
exercises
  Being the Future You, 161
  Clearing Using "The River," 171
  Clearing Your Energy Using a Body Proxy, 165, 168–69, 171
  Connect to a Celestial Being, 149
  Connect with a Power Animal, 144
  Despacho Ceremony, 176
  Dial It Up or Down, 173
  Doing a Focused Clearing, 171
  Drawing a New "Story," 113
  Earth, Sky, Heart Meditation, 175
  Engaging with the Elements, 71
  Feeling and Working with Your Energy Field, 120
  Hall of Contracts, 59–60, 165, 184, 188
  Invocation for Your Journey, 189
  Journaling with the Four 'A's, 87
  Journey and Dialogue to Gain Awareness and Increase Intuition, 130
  Ritual to Eliminate the Negative, 172
  Running the Colors, 123, 187
  Sand Painting, 178–79
expansion, 98–99, 101

Four 'A's (also see Act, Allow, Affirm, Aware), 191

Four Winds Society, 17, 19, 27, 58, 102, 144, 158, 168
Healing the Light Body, 23, 25, 148

gratitude, 57, 61–62, 97, 99, 107, 165, 167, 176–80
gut distress, 174, 186

helpers, 56–57, 59, 137–39, 143
ancestors, 41, 93, 139–40
angels, 142
ascended masters, 142
dragons, 136–37, 139, 142
elementals, 141
Higher Self, 83, 103, 107, 139–40,184
nature spirits, 139, 141
power animal, 56, 105, 139–40, 144

intention, 56, 84, 86, 92, 98–99, 101, 107, 154–60, 163
intuition, 84, 118, 130

joint pain, 69, 187–88

life force, 5, 47, 97, 99, 164, 171, 174
light body (see luminous energy body)
luminous energy field/body, 19–20, 46, 86, 95, 107, 110, 119

Maximum Medicine, 37–38, 48, 82, 88, 110, 118, 181
Maximum Medicine Mindfulness Matrix, 88
Medicine Wheel
Wheel of the Four Directions, 63, 66, 91

Wheel of the Four Elements, 63, 66, 68
Wheel of the Four Perspectives, 63, 73
Wheel of the Four Inner Actions, 63, 82, 88, 118, 164
Wheel of the Four Inner Tasks, 63, 82, 84, 88, 118
meditation (see exercises)
mesa, 64, 165–72, 178

perspectives
emotional, 71, 74, 77–79, 89
energetic, 75–76, 78–80
literal, 73, 77–78
spiritual, 75, 78–79, 94
power, 63, 88–89, 140
power animal, 56, 85, 104, 139–41, 143–44, 146, 148, 152, 166

ritual, 42, 84, 86, 108, 125, 164, 172, 174, 180

sacred space, 21, 56, 89, 104–105, 165, 175
sacred vortex, 165
shamanic healing, 22, 38
shamanic practitioner, 24, 40, 45, 58
shamanism, 13, 23–24, 27, 34, 39, 42, 47–48, 67, 140

transformation, 98–99, 103

universal energy field, 23, 27, 41
universal matrix, 20, 23–24
universe, 20, 41, 49, 107, 109, 138, 152, 158, 177

Wise One, 129, 132–33, 139, 150, 184

Acknowledgments

I would like to acknowledge some people who were invaluable in bringing this book forward.

Drs. Carl Greer, Patrice Fields, and **Georgia Herrera** – From these powerful mystics and healers I honed my spirituality and healing skills. I literally would not be who I am today without the guidance of these amazing teachers.

My spiritual community – The sacred container we hold has sustained, nourished, and propelled me forward into expansion. You are my heart.

Dr. Pat Baccili and **Jesica Henderson** – These women held the vision of what I could achieve, even in the absence of my future sight. They also brought me into the world of communication, in forms I had never tried before. I owe you guys.

CC Treadway and **Lizzie Rose**, in concert with the Sisters of the Red Rose, the Advanced Channeling Group, and the Weavers of Time – My spiritual classmates, who walked with me on my many journeys, I have loved traveling with you.

The Four Winds Society and my shaman classmates – I cut my shamanic teeth studying in the Light Body curriculum, and in doing so, woke up a dormant but potent part of myself. I offer my deepest gratitude.

Nancy Peske – I am very appreciative of her masterful editorial skills, ability to organize, use the perfect phrase, and hold the big-picture view, all of which have lent substance and finesse to this book.

About the Author

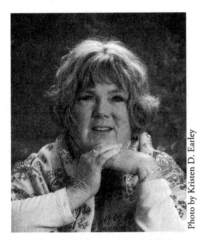

Photo by Kristen D. Earley

Dr. Sharon Martin holds a doctorate in Physiology and worked as a research scientist and teaching faculty at Emory University School of Medicine in Atlanta, Georgia. Subsequently, she trained at and graduated from Johns Hopkins School of Medicine in Baltimore, Maryland, and finished a medical residency in Internal Medicine. During the last year of her Internal Medicine residency, Dr. Martin served as Chief Resident. Dr. Martin continues to hold membership in the American College of Physicians, the national organization for Internal Medicine physicians. She is certified by the national American Board of Internal Medicine.

Dr. Martin is a certified graduate of the Healing the Light Body curriculum of the Four Winds Society, a premier training program in shamanic energy medicine. She is currently the medical director of a rural health clinic in south-central Pennsylvania. She also is the host of two radio shows, "*Maximum Medicine*" and "*Sacred Magic*," which air on the internationally renowned syndicated network *Transformation Talk Radio*.

For more information visit: **www.drsharonmartin.com**

FINDHORN PRESS

Life-Changing Books

Learn more about us and our books at
www.findhornpress.com

For information on the Findhorn Foundation:
www.findhorn.org